ESSENTIAL 101 TIPS

# HOMEOPATHY

Dr Andrew Lockie

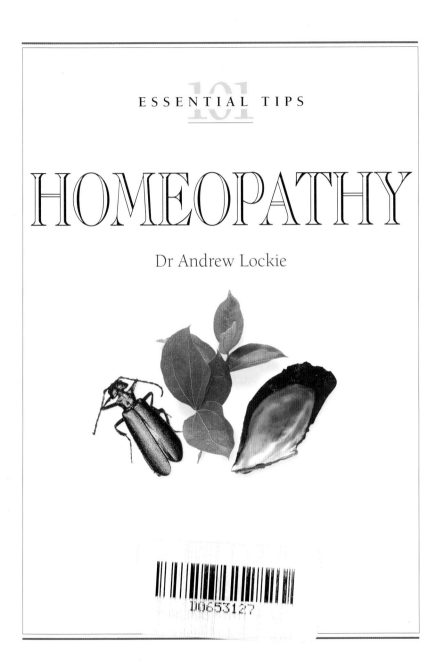

D0653127

DORLING KINDERSLEY
LONDON, NEW YORK, AUCKLAND, DELHI,
JOHANNESBURG, MUNICH, PARIS, SYDNEY

DK www.dk.com

**Editor** Bella Pringle
**Art Editor** Colin Walton
**DTP Designer** Robert Campbell
**Senior Editor** Peter Jones
**Senior Art Editor** Heather McCarry
**Managing Editor** Anna Kruger
**Managing Art Editor** Stephen Knowlden
**Production Controller** Louise Daly

First published in Great Britain in 2000 by
Dorling Kindersley Limited, 9 Henrietta Street, London WC2E 8PS

A CIP catalogue record for this book is available from the British Library

ISBN 0 7513 2002 1

Text film output by Colourscan
Reproduced by Colourscan
Printed by Wing King Tong, Hong Kong

# ESSENTIAL TIPS

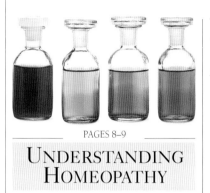

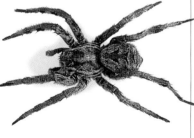

# VEGETABLE REMEDIES

# MINERAL REMEDIES

# USING THE REMEDIES

# UNDERSTANDING HOMEOPATHY

## 1 WHAT IS HOMEOPATHY?

Homeopathy is a holistic form of medicine where diagnosis takes into account the individual physical and emotional characteristics of the patient. Remedies are chosen to match the symptoms as closely as possible, and so may be different for patients with the same affliction. The emphasis is on prevention and a person's involvement with their own cure. Homeopathic remedies help the body to help itself. There is not always a quick cure. Homeopaths categorize each individual into constitutional types to assess which remedies will best suit them.

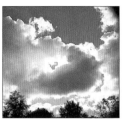
△ GENERAL FACTORS
*The weather conditions, the seasons, temperature, and time of day may all have an effect on physical and mental well-being.*

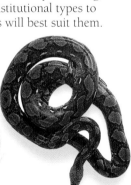

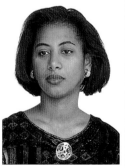

△ FOOD PREFERENCES
*The foods an individual likes and dislikes are an important part of assessing constitutional types.*

△ FEARS
*Tangible fears, such as fear of snakes, and intangible fears, such as fear of failure, are considered.*

△ PERSONALITY
*People are categorized according to emotional characteristics, such as optimism or irritability.*

# 2 THE ORIGINS OF HOMEOPATHY

The founder of homeopathy in the late 18th century was a German doctor, Samuel Hahnemann. He believed that what could cause disease could also cure in tiny doses. He demonstrated his theory when he dosed himself with quinine, the cure for malaria, and developed malaria-like symptoms. This principle that like can cure like, first postulated by Hippocrates in the fifth century BC, remains central to homeopathy.

▽ BELLADONNA
*Hahnemann used deadly nightshade, which is poisonous, to cure scarlet fever.*

# 3 MODERN HOMEOPATHY

Hahnemann pioneered a way of diluting remedies whereby they acted faster and more effectively than a concentrated solution. This method, known as succussing, involves vigorous shaking of the remedy. The potency of a remedy is related to its dilution (*see Tip 11*).

Later followers identified certain constitutional types, based on the observation that people with similar personalities and body shapes tend to suffer from the same types of disease.

REMEDIES ▷
*Most usually available as lactose tablets, modern remedies are also found in liquid and ointment form.*

# 4 COMPARISON WITH ORTHODOX MEDICINE

In orthodox medicine, the disease is treated rather than the whole person, or their, perhaps unique, symptoms. Homeopathy takes into account underlying causes as well as the symptoms of a disease before prescribing a remedy.

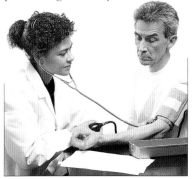

△ TREATING SYMPTOMS
*In orthodox medicine, it is the disease itself rather than the individual that is treated.*

# HOMEOPATHY IN ACTION

## 5 VITAL FORCE

Hahnemann called the body's own healing energy the "vital force", reasoning that this force was what enabled such tiny amounts of remedy to cause healing. If the force is disturbed by stress, poor diet, or lack of exercise, then it cannot do its job of maintaining a healthy body and illness results. The symptoms of illness are the outward manifestation of the vital force's attempt to redress imbalance and restore order.

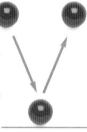

△ STRONG FORCE
*Stresses that beset a strong vital force are deflected quickly; the body recuperates fast to keep good health.*

△ WEAK FORCE
*If the vital force is weak, the body does not have the energy to fight illness.*

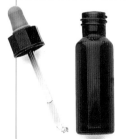

BACH RESCUE REMEDY
*This tincture is a good treatment for worry or panic, nervousness, and trembling.*

## 6 TREATING YOURSELF

Self-prescribing homeopathic remedies is a safe and effective method of treating most minor, acute complaints, such as a cold. The remedies can also play an important part in first aid after accidents. If an illness recurs or symptoms persist, it may be an indication of a chronic illness for which you need professional help. If your homeopath is not medically trained, it is wise to continue taking advice from your healthcare practitioner. In homeopathy, maintaining a healthy lifestyle, coping well with stress, and adopting a strong emotional outlook all play an important part in the prevention of illness.

# 7 FINDING QUALIFIED HOMEOPATHS

The increasing popularity of homeopathy has made choosing a practitioner much easier. Many countries around the world now consider homeopathy a viable alternative to orthodox medicine and pharmaceutical drugs. India, some countries in Europe (particularly the UK, Germany, and France), Canada and the USA, Australia, and South America all show increasing practice of homeopathy. If you cannot find a homeopath through personal recommendation, then national regulatory bodies should supply a list of homeopaths in your area.

# 8 CONSULTING A HOMEOPATH

On your first visit you will be categorized into a constitutional type by an assessment of your appearance, symptoms, food likes and dislikes, bodily functions, fears, and lifestyle.

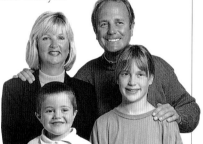

HOMEOPATHS CAN HELP THE WHOLE FAMILY

# 9 SOURCE OF REMEDIES

Remedies are made from plant, animal, or mineral extracts, diluted in varying degrees. Sources range from toxic snake venom to foods, such as oats or onions. Some of the sources have been used undiluted for many years in orthodox medicine or herbalism, and have been homeopathically proved by the principle of like curing like.

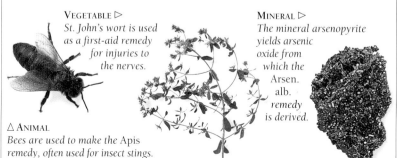

VEGETABLE ▷
*St. John's wort is used as a first-aid remedy for injuries to the nerves.*

MINERAL ▷
*The mineral arsenopyrite yields arsenic oxide from which the Arsen. alb. remedy is derived.*

△ ANIMAL
*Bees are used to make the Apis remedy, often used for insect stings.*

# 10 HOW REMEDIES ARE MADE

Making remedies is a very precise process. The raw material is dissolved in nine parts alcohol and one part distilled water, left to stand for several days, and shaken occasionally. This mix is then strained through a press, resulting in a liquid called the "mother tincture". To make the remedy, the tincture is repeatedly diluted in an alcohol/water mix. Between every stage of dilution, the tincture is shaken vigorously. Drops of this tincture are then added to tablets.

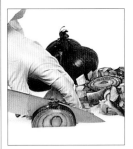

1 Fresh onions are thoroughly washed and some of the outer skin removed before being coarsely chopped.

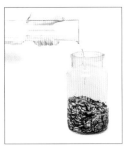

2 The chopped onions are put into a large sealable glass jar. An alcohol/water mixture is poured onto the onions.

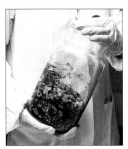

3 The jar is then sealed with an airtight lid and allowed to stand for up to four weeks, and shaken occasionally.

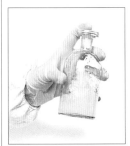

5 One drop of mother tincture is added to 99 drops of an alcohol/water mixture and shaken vigorously (succussed).

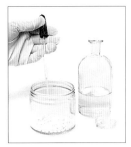

6 The mixture is succussed and diluted repeatedly. Drops of the potentized remedy are added to lactose tablets.

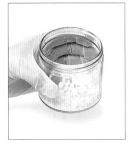

7 The lactose tablets are swirled around to make sure that each one is impregnated with the potentized remedy.

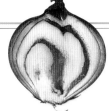

**RED ONION**
*A tincture of red onion is the basis for the Allium remedy, prepared below.*

# 11 POTENCY OF REMEDIES

The potency of a remedy describes its dilution, or strength, and is measured on one of two scales. In the decimal scale (x), the dilution factor is one part of tincture to ten parts alcohol and water, while in the centesimal scale (c), it is 1 to 100. The number of a remedy shows how many times it has been diluted and succussed.

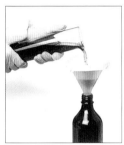

4 The resulting liquid is strained through a press, and this "mother tincture" is then strained into a dark bottle.

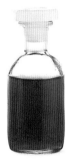

**3C STRENGTH**
*This remedy has been diluted and succussed only three times.*

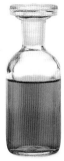

**6C STRENGTH**
*This remedy has been diluted and succussed only six times.*

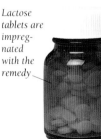

*Lactose tablets are impregnated with the remedy*

8 The tablets are then placed in an airtight dark glass bottle and stored away from the effects of direct sunlight.

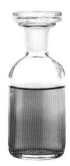

**12C STRENGTH**
*One part of tincture to a hundred parts alcohol and water succussed 12 times.*

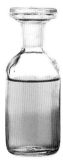

**30C STRENGTH**
*This has been diluted 30 times, which makes it the strongest remedy seen here.*

# ASSESSING YOUR HEALTH

## 12 HOMEOPATHIC TYPES

As the basis of a homeopathic assessment, a practitioner collects a wealth of information about a patient's physical condition, as well as mental and emotional states, and life in general. An individual's unique adaptations to their own surroundings and their idiosyncratic ways are accepted and respected for making an individual what they are. Every person is regarded as the product of their physical and mental well-being or ill-health, genetic inheritance, and also daily experience. By arranging people into types based on their make-up, experienced homeopaths match the remedy to person. The name given is that of the remedy that matches closest.

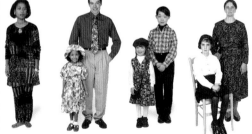

△ ASSESSING YOUR HOMEOPATHIC TYPE
*Despite the individualistic nature of homeopathic assessment and treatment, people are grouped according to their physical attributes, and mental and emotional traits.*

**ARGENT. NIT.**
*Individuals of this type are driven: they think, talk, and act rapidly. They are extrovert, cheerful, and impressionable but are prone to lose their tempers, or become anxious. Weak areas include sensitive digestion, the nerves, and mucous membranes.*

**ARSEN. ALB.**
*These are restless, tense, ambitious individuals who are perfectionists by nature and intolerant of disorder. Pessimistic, they need constant reassurance. Illness brings rapid physical and mental exhaustion; weak areas include the respiratory and digestive tracts.*

**CALC. CARB.**
*Quiet, cautious, and very sensitive, these types are outwardly strong and stoical looking. Generally they are healthy, and when ill become depressed and introspective. They can be obsessive. Weak areas include bones, teeth, bowels, and skin.*

### GRAPHITES
*These types are anxious, timid, and indecisive. They are slow to react to external stimuli and are prone to frequent mood changes. More physically than intellectually orientated, weak areas are the skin and metabolism.*

### LYCOPODIUM
*This type tends to be intellectual with a conservative outlook. Their self-possession belies a strong sense of insecurity, and they are resistant to change. They are intolerant of illness. Weak areas centre on digestive problems with excess bloating and wind.*

### NUX VOMICA
*Highly strung, energetic, competitive achievers, these workaholic personalities work and play hard, thriving on challenges. Critical of others, they readily explode in anger. Their lifestyle tends to affect weak areas including stomach, bowels, and liver.*

### SEPIA
*Mainly women, Sepia types tend to adopt a martyr's role. They are opinionated and hate to be contradicted. They are independent, yet can feel overwhelmed by their responsibilities. Sepia is chiefly linked with the treatment of hormone-related ailments.*

### IGNATIA
*Most Ignatia types are women. They are artistic, sensitive, and highly strung, with a tendency to overreact. They find it difficult to express their emotions. Weak areas include their mental health and the nervous system.*

### MERC. SOL.
*Introverted and closed, Merc. sol types seem detached and arrogant, but this conceals strong emotions. They need order and stability. Weak areas include the blood and mucous membranes. Mouth ulcers, abscesses, fever, and swollen glands are common.*

### PHOS.
*These types are expressive and affectionate, often artistic, although their enthusiasm can be intense and short-lived, and they may rapidly exhaust their energy when under pressure or ill. Weak areas of the body include chest, lungs, and digestion.*

### SILICEA
*These types are tenacious and stubborn, yet appear fragile and sensitive. They lack physical and mental stamina, and can be obsessive about detail. Their outlook is limited by fear of failure. Weak areas include the digestive and nervous systems.*

### LACHESIS
*Individuals of this type live life intensely, with a sense of physical and mental congestion – being confined is difficult and they may resist commitment. The nervous system plus the blood and circulation are weak areas.*

### NATRUM MUR.
*Extremely sensitive and refined, Natrum mur. types are often women. They are serious and conscientious, easily hurt by criticism, yet are idealistic and inflexible. Either pear-shaped or with a square build, their weak areas include the digestive tract and blood.*

### PULSATILLA
*Pulsatilla types are usually women. Shy, gentle, and kind, they are not assertive and avoid confrontation, and tend to be swayed by emotion rather than thought. Their symptoms are changeable; weak areas of the body include the veins and stomach.*

### SULPHUR
*Imaginative and inventive, Sulphur types are inept on a practical level, living life at an intellectual level. Pedantic and egotistical, they have a strong desire for recognition and expend a lot of energy on ideas and speculation. Weak areas include the circulation.*

# 13 EFFECTS OF DIET

It is important to eat a healthy, balanced diet to provide the nutrients required for good health, avoiding too many cholesterol-rich and refined foods. Some conditions, such as diabetes and heart disease, are linked to the over-consumption of certain food types, and many ailments can be prevented or improved by altering the diet, and taking extra nutrients in the form of supplements. Knowing a person's food preferences helps the trained homeopath to assess their overall health, and also tells them about that person's constitutional type.

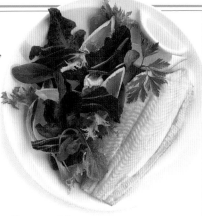

**BALANCED MEAL**
*Wholefoods such as salads, vegetables, bread, and pasta should form the bulk of a balanced diet. Fish, dairy products, and meat need each only be eaten twice a week.*

# 14 DAILY EXERCISE

Other factors used by homeopaths to help determine a person's constitutional type are their physical appearance, and their level of indoor and outdoor activity. Some people are energetic by nature, while others are sluggish and lack stamina. The human body is designed for muscular activity, however, and does not function properly without it. Homeopaths therefore encourage fitness and regular exercise.

*Exercise benefits the heart*

**HEALTHY CYCLING**
*Cycling to work is an excellent way of building strenuous exercise into your daily routine. It is best to start any exercise plan slowly and build up gradually.*

## 15 ENVIRONMENTAL FACTORS

The weather, the seasons, the time of day, and temperature changes influence people in different ways. Noting how these environmental factors affect someone generally, as well as their influence on specific illnesses, can significantly assist the homeopath to determine a person's constitutional type. A person suffering pain in the knee may feel better for a warm compress applied to the affected area, but may feel worse for heat generally. Whether someone finds the approach of a thunderstorm relaxing, or headache-inducing, for example, how he or she reacts to sea air, and how easily he or she wakes in the morning, all aid an understanding of that person's constitutional type.

## 16 THE IMPORTANCE OF SLEEP

Lack of sleep is a very important contributory cause of stress, and can also lead to illness. Your sleep patterns, dream content, and usual sleeping position may all be taken into account by a homeopath.

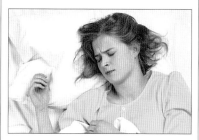

REJUVENATION THROUGH SLEEP
*Many people are exhausted from inadequate rest and sleep, either due to physical or emotional stress. Follow a routine for going to bed to help insomnia.*

## 17 COPING WITH STRESS

Stress can be defined as anything that puts pressure on the body's systems. A certain amount of stress is good: performance and efficiency both improve. When levels are too high, fatigue sets in, possibly followed by illness. Short-term stress is relatively easy to deal with: any activity that you find relaxing and that calms your mind will help dissipate stress. For more severe cases, techniques such as yoga, meditation, and t'ai chi can all be helpful. A positive mental attitude helps to control stress and confront it head on.

MEDITATION
*Deep breathing and meditating can help calm the mind and reduce stress.*

*Try not to dwell on your problems*

17

# ANIMAL REMEDIES

## 18  APIS / HONEY BEE

(*Apis mellifica*) Honey bees provide a range of medicinal substances: the whole bee, honey, beeswax, resin from the hive, royal jelly, and pollen are all used. The *Apis* remedy is commonly used in homeopathy for inflammation with burning, stinging pain, especially where the skin is itchy, swollen, and very sensitive to touch. It is also used for urinary tract infections, fluid retention, and allergic conditions in the eyes, mouth, and throat.

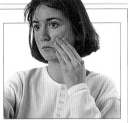

**CALMING INSECT STINGS**
*Use* Apis *where the area around a sting is hot, red, and swollen. Take 30c every 15 minutes, for six doses.*

**KEY USES**
• *Burning, stinging pain that is worse for heat and better for cold.*
• *Tight, blister-like swellings sensitive to light pressure.*
• *Fever without thirst and a dry skin.*
• *Symptoms that start on the right side of the body.*

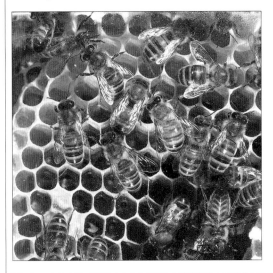

◁ ***Honey bees*** *The* Apis *remedy is made from the whole bee, including the sting. Honey, pollen, and royal jelly are also used.*

# 19 CANTHARIS / SPANISH FLY

(*Cantharis vesicatoria*) Perhaps best known as an aphrodisiac in love potions, the homeopathic remedy from spanish fly is given for complaints with burning symptoms. The bright green beetle secretes an irritant substance called cantharidin, which is a powerful poison if taken in large doses. It attacks the urinary tract and causes violent vomiting and burning pain. *Cantharis* is used to treat severe cystitis, and other urinary tract infections, as well as scalds and burns. Mental problems eased by *Cantharis* homeopathic remedy include excessive desire for sexual intercourse, fits of rage, severe anxiety, and irritability leading to violence.

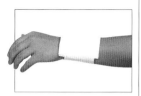

**TREATING BURNS**
*If a burn is bigger than the palm of a hand, consult a doctor immediately. Apply cold compresses and take 30c of Cantharsis every 15 minutes, for six doses.*

*Beetle secretes irritant called cantharidin*

*Actual size*

△ **SPANISH FLIES**
*These insects, mainly to be found in Spain and southern France, are the source of the Cantharis remedy, used for aliments with burning, stinging pain.*

**KEY USES**
• *Ailments characterized by burning, stinging pain and a great thirst but no desire to drink, such as urinary tract infections.*
• *Burns and stings.*
• *Conditions that tend to worsen rapidly.*
• *Mental problems, such as rage and deep anxiety.*

*Whole beetle is used to make remedy*

△ **LYTTA VESICATORIA**
*These poisonous and highly irritant bright green beetles have been used medicinally since ancient times.*

# 20 LACHESIS / BUSHMASTER SNAKE

(*Lachesis muta*) If a bite from this snake enters a vein directly, it can be fatal. Superficial snake bites cause profuse bleeding and also blood-poisoning. The *Lachesis* remedy made from the venom acts mainly on the blood and circulation and is used to treat engorged, throbbing veins. It is also helpful when the skin on the extremities appears purple-blue due to circulatory problems. A weak heart; a rapid, weak, irregular pulse; palpitations; angina; and difficulty in breathing are all eased by this remedy, as are menopausal and premenstrual symptoms.`

**DRIED VENOM**
*The remedy made from venom is used for wounds that bleed freely.*

**BUSHMASTER SNAKE ▷**
*This snake is an aggressive hunter: bites can be fatal.*

*Also given for fainting in menopause*

*Venom is "milked" from live snake*

◁ **MENOPAUSAL SYMPTOMS**
*This key remedy for menopausal women is given for hot flushes. The dosage is 30c taken every 12 hours for up to 7 days.*

**KEY USES**
• *Circulatory problems and vascular complaints.*
• *Menopausal and premenstrual symptoms.*
• *Slow-to-heal wounds.*
• *Left-sided ailments that tend to be worse for suppressing emotions.*
• *Throat complaints.*

# 21 SEPIA / CUTTLEFISH

(*Sepia officinalis*) Medicinally, cuttlefish ink was used in ancient times to treat kidney stones and gonorrhea. *Sepia* acts on the uterus, ovaries, and vagina, and is given for painful or heavy menstruation, hot flushes in menopause, thrush, emotional and physical symptoms in pregnancy, and helps women who suffer pain during sexual intercourse. Ailments that are accompanied by exhaustion, indigestion from milk and fatty foods, headaches with nausea, dizziness, and varicose veins all benefit from *Sepia*.

**KEY USES**
• *Women's complaints, especially conditions related to hormone imbalance, such as PMS (premenstrual syndrome) and menopause.*
• *Ailments accompanied by exhaustion.*

*Often changes colour to blend in*

**CUTTLEFISH ▷**
*The remedy is made from pure pigments in the brownish-black ink it squirts for protection.*

# 22 TARENTULA / WOLF SPIDER

(*Tarentula hispanica*) Unlike its South American relative, this European tarentula is not dangerous to humans. The whole live spider is used to make a remedy to treat disorders of the nervous system, as well as heart disorders, such as angina and heart disease. In women, it is given for ovarian disease and sensitive, itchy genitalia.

**KEY USES**
• *Extreme physical and mental restlessness.*
• *Heart disorders.*
• *Ovarian disease.*
• *Sensitive, itchy genitalia in women.*
• *Complaints where person tends to roll from side to side for relief.*

*Whole live spider is used in remedy*

**WOLF SPIDER**
*The spider's common name stems from the fact that it chases prey, rather than catching it in a web.*

# VEGETABLE REMEDIES

## 23 ACONITE / MONKSHOOD

*(Aconitum napellus)* This deadly plant has been used throughout history as an arrow poison in hunting. Hahnemann and his successors used it extensively as a homeopathic remedy for fevers and sudden complaints with severe pain, which until then had been treated by blood-letting. The remedy is usually needed at the onset of colds and coughs, and eye, ear, and throat complaints, with symptoms of inflammation and infection. *Aconite* is also given for fear with associated restlessness, for example, panic attacks with palpitations, numbness, and tingling in the body.

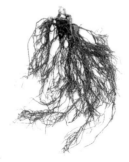

◁△ MONKSHOOD
*This plant is highly toxic; the root contains nine times more poison than its leaves.*

### KEY USES
• *Complaints that come on suddenly and acutely, often due to shock or fright, or are brought on by abrupt changes in weather conditions.*
• *Fear and shock, and a fear of dying when ill, especially for women who fear death during labour.*
• *Burning pain and numbness in the body.*

# 24 ALLIUM / ONION

*(Allium cepa)* Among the world's oldest plants, and long renowned for its healing properties, the onion contains a volatile oil that stimulates the tear glands and the mucous membranes of the upper respiratory tract, causing the eyes and nose to water. The homeopathic remedy made from the red onion bulb is used to treat illnesses in which the main symptoms include streaming eyes and nasal discharge, such as hay fever and colds. It is also used to treat any burning sensation or neuralgic pain that alternates from side to side, usually from left to right.

*Papery outer layers are discarded*

**KEY USES**
• *Burning sensation or neuralgic pain.*
•*Symptoms or pains that alternate from side to side, usually moving from the left to the right.*
• *Complaints with a burning, streaming discharge, especially from the eyes and nose.*
• *Laryngitis, hoarseness, and coughs.*

*Fresh red bulb is used to make remedy*

△ **RED ONION**
*Onions cause burning tears and the remedy is used to treat complaints that cause the eyes to sting or water.*

◁ **HAY FEVER**
*A dose of 6c taken for up to ten doses benefits hay fever sufferers with a burning nasal discharge.*

*Nasal discharge moves from left to right*

# 25 ARNICA

(*Arnica montana*) Arnica was well known to country people as a remedy for muscular aches and bruises. It is now used internally in homeopathic doses for shock, to promote the healing of damaged tissues, and to help control bleeding. Used internally or externally, arnica aids joint and muscle problems such as osteoarthritis, aching muscles from unaccustomed exercise, cramps, bruises, and strains. It is also given internally for eczema, boils, concussion, and black eyes as well as for eyestrain and fever, where the head feels hot, but the body is cold.

ARNICA ▷
*In orthodox medicine,
Arnica montana has been
used to treat dysentery, gout,
malaria, and rheumatism.*

*Remedy is
made from
whole fresh
plant in flower*

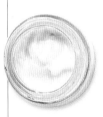

△ ARNICA CREAM
*This is used externally for
bruises and sprains, but
not on broken skin because
it may cause a rash*

KEY USES
• *An excellent first aid
remedy.*
• *Shock, pain, bruising,
and other injuries, and
bleeding caused by
accidental injuries.*
• *Emotional shock, for
example following
sudden bereavement.*

◁ ROOT
*The fresh arnica root,
which grows on the
mountains of Europe,
is popular with
mountain climbers.*

*The root is chewed to
relieve aching muscles.*

# 26 BELLADONNA / DEADLY NIGHTSHADE

(*Atropa belladonna*) Allegedly used in witchcraft in
the Middle Ages, and in orthodox medicine for spasms,
nausea, and vertigo, *Belladonna* was proved as a
homeopathic remedy for Hahnemann
when he used it to treat scarlet fever.
Aside from infections and inflammations
with sudden onset, it is used to help
pounding headaches, boils, fits, labour
pain, and restless sleep.

*Fresh leaves
and flowers
are used for
remedy*

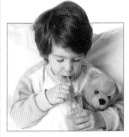

△ **RELIEVING FEVER**
*It is given to children
suffering from a high fever,
and to ease teething pain.*

**KEY USES**
• *Acute complaints with a
sudden and violent onset,
and throbbing pain and
flushing due to increased
blood circulation.*
• *High fever with dilated
pupils and staring eyes.*
• *Ailments where there is
extreme sensitivity to
light, noise, and touch.*

△ **BELLADONNA**
*Although all plant parts are
poisonous, it has been used
throughout history to treat
infection and inflammation.*

# 27 BRYONIA / BRYONY

(*Bryonia alba*) Acute
conditions that develop slowly
such as coughs, flu, and
headaches, and ailments
characterized by dryness of the
mouth, lips, chest, or eyes are
treated with *Bryonia*. The fresh
root is very poisonous: death
is caused from inflammation
of the digestive tract. When ill,
people who need *Bryonia* are
reluctant to move or speak.

**KEY USES**
• *Slow-starting
conditions where
pain is felt on even
slight movement.*
• *Problems with
dry mouth, lips,
eyes, and chest.*

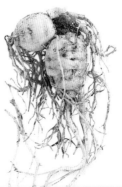

◁ **FRESH ROOT**
*To make the
remedy, fresh roots
are chopped and
pounded to a pulp.*

# 28 CHINA

(*China officinalis*) Made from Peruvian bark, this was the first substance that Hahnemann tested on himself. He noted that in large doses, quinine (extracted from the bark) causes similar symptoms to malaria, which it cures. Today, *China* remedies treat symptoms such as exhaustion, as well as headaches, neuralgia, convulsions, dizziness, haemorrhages, and nosebleeds.

*Bark must be dried before it can be used*

**KEY USES**
• *Nervous exhaustion resulting from debilitating conditions.*
• *Weakness that results from loss of bodily fluids through sweating, diarrhoea, or vomiting.*

◁ **DRIED BARK**
*The bark comes from the evergreen Cinchona tree, which grows in tropical forests.*

# 29 CIMIC. / BLACK COHOSH

(*Cimicifuga racemosa*) This remedy acts on the nerves and muscles of the uterus, so it is largely a women's remedy, used for menstrual symptoms (congestion in the head and cramps), early miscarriage, and common pregnancy complaints such as nausea and sleeplessness. Post-natal depression and menopausal symptoms are also helped, as are neck stiffness that causes headaches and emotional symptoms from hormonal imbalance.

**KEY USES**
• *Complaints related to menstruation, pregnancy, birth, and menopause.*
• *Headaches.*
• *Sighing and sadness.*

**BLACK COHOSH** ▷
*Native Americans used the root as a cure for rattle-snake bites, and for menstrual and labour pain. They also chewed it to alleviate depression and as a sedative.*

*Remedy made from fresh root and rhizome*

## 30 COLOCYNTHIS / BITTER APPLE

*(Cucumis colocynthis)* The main conditions treated with *Colocynthis* are characterized by colicky or neuralgic pain caused by suppressed anger. The remedy is effective for headaches, facial neuralgia, stomach pain with nausea or vomiting, and abdominal pain with diarrhoea. Nerve pain around the kidneys or ovaries, gout, sciatica (pain along the sciatic nerve), rheumatism, and dizziness associated with rheumatism in the neck, are all helped by *Colocynthis*.

△ BITTER APPLE
*The* Colocynthis *remedy is made from the dried fruit, seeds discarded, which is powdered.*

**KEY USES**
• *Extreme anger and indignation that causes colicky or neuralgic pain.*
• *Digestive upsets.*
• *Headaches associated with anger or embarrassment.*

## 31 DROSERA / SUNDEW

*(Drosera rotundifolia)* This is mainly a cough remedy, used to treat violent coughs that are spasmodic, deep, rasping, and hollow. In the acute stages the cough can end in gagging, vomiting, and nosebleeds. When ill, people who need this remedy are restless, obstinate, anxious when alone, and find it hard to concentrate. Other symptoms *Drosera* benefits are a hoarse voice, stiffness, and inflexible ankles.

◁ SUNDEW
*The whole fresh plant in flower is used for the remedy. The plant juice is caustic, and acts on the respiratory system.*

**KEY USES**
• *Violent, hollow-sounding coughs that are worse after midnight, such as whooping cough.*
• *Growing pains and bone pain.*
• *Restlessness and obstinacy.*

## 32 EUPHRASIA / EYEBRIGHT

(*Euphrasia officinale*) Eye complaints such as conjunctivitis, blepharitis (inflammation of the eyelids), iritis (inflammation of the iris), dimmed vision, intolerance of bright light, sticky mucus or blisters on the cornea, and dry eyes in menopause all benefit from this remedy. Colds and hay fever with hot, red cheeks and watery catarrh are also helped. In addition, it is used to treat bursting headaches, constipation, and the early stages of measles.

*Whole fresh plant in flower used for remedy*

**KEY USES**
• *Eye complaints characterized by watery, burning, stinging eyes.*
• *Eye injuries or inflammation.*
• *Hay fever with an irritating eye discharge, but clear nasal discharge.*

EYEBRIGHT ▷
*This plant has long been used as a cure for eye complaints: it was first mentioned as an eye medicine in 1305. It is still used by herbalists.*

## 33 GELSEMIUM / YELLOW JASMINE

(*Gelsemium sempervirens*) This remedy mainly affects the brain and spinal cord, the motor nerves, the muscles, eyelids, and mucous membranes. It helps the following: headaches that intensify with movement or bright light, a sore scalp due to nerve inflammation, muscle pain associated with fever, and nervous disorders, such as multiple sclerosis. It is given for fears and phobias that are accompanied by trembling.

**YELLOW JASMINE** ▽
*This climbing plant causes paralysis if taken in large doses. The remedy is made from the fresh root.*

*Fresh root is aromatic*

**KEY USES**
• *Conditions of the nervous system.*
• *Headaches and eye problems.*
• *Colds and flu.*
• *Fears and phobias.*
• *Infections with feverish symptoms.*

# 34 HAMAMELIS / WITCH HAZEL

(*Hamamelis virginiana*) The binding and contracting properties of the bark make this an excellent remedy for internal and external bleeding. The remedy is used for weak and inflamed veins and bleeding, bruising, and soreness due to injury, nosebleeds, weakness from blood loss caused by a burst inflamed vein, and painful, bloodshot or black eyes. It is also used in the treatment of depression.

**KEY USES**
- *Weak inflamed veins, and bleeding.*
- *Bruising and soreness.*
- *Nosebleeds.*
- *Weakness caused by blood loss from burst vein.*
- *Depression.*

*Only the outer layer of the fresh root is used*

**HAMAMELIS ROOTS AND BARK △▷**
*The outer layer of the fresh root and the bark of the twigs are chopped and pounded to a pulp to make the homeopathic remedy.*

# 35 HYPERICUM / ST. JOHN'S WORT

(*Hypericum perforatum*) *Hypericum* is the most important remedy for injuries to any part of the body with a high concentration of nerve endings, such as the fingers, toes, spine, eyes, lips, nailbeds, and head. It is an excellent first aid remedy for any kind of puncture wound, for example from nails, splinters, or bites, and crushed fingers and toes. It is also used for asthma that is worse in cold, damp weather.

**ST. JOHN'S WORT ▷**
*The whole fresh plant in flower is used. A hypericum tincture is good first aid for cuts, scrapes, and grazes.*

**KEY USES**
- *Injuries to the nerves with nerve pain.*
- *Severe shooting pain that travels upwards. It can also treat asthma.*
- *Effects of head injuries.*
- *Asthma worse in fog.*

# 36 IGNATIA / ST. IGNATIUS' BEAN

*(Ignatia amara)* This remedy is given by homeopaths to treat emotional problems: it is a key remedy for bereavement with mood swings, hysteria, and insomnia. Other emotional states it relieves include self-pity, sudden tearfulness, depression, and worry. It is effective for headaches, and for ailments with contradictory symptoms, such as nausea and vomiting that is better for eating. It also benefits tickly coughs, fever and chills that induce thirst, fainting in confined conditions, and upper abdominal pain.

*Seeds contain the poison strychnine*

◁ **IGNATIA SEEDS**
*The seeds of this large East Asian tree are separated from the pulp surrounding them, then powdered to make the homeopathic remedy.*

**KEY USES**
- *Emotional problems.*
- *Acute grief caused by bereavement or broken relationships.*
- *Headaches.*
- *Coughs and sore throats.*
- *Changeable symptoms.*

# 37 IPECAC. / IPECACUANHA

*(Cephaelis ipecacuanha)* Physical symptoms helped by *Ipecac.* include persistent nausea with pale face, hot or cold sweats and clamminess, and nausea associated with migraines. Stomach ailments accompanied by a weak pulse, lack of thirst, and fainting also benefit, as do breathing difficulties, such as asthma and fitful coughing leading to choking.

**KEY USES**
- *Constant nausea, with or without vomiting.*
- *Difficulty in breathing and a feeling of suffocation.*
- *Profuse, bright red bleeding.*

△ **IPECAC.**
*The root of this rainforest perennial is collected while the plant is in flower, and then dried to make the homeopathic remedy. It is mainly used for nausea and vomiting.*

# 38 LEDUM / WILD ROSEMARY

(*Ledum palustre*) As well as first aid applications for injuries or stings where there is severe bruising, *Ledum* is given for rheumatic pain; stiff, painful joints; pain in the toes due to gout; and painful, swollen, and stiff tendons. Symptoms of all complaints are eased by applying cold compresses to the affected part, but are worse at night, for warmth and touch. People needing the remedy prefer to be left alone when ill.

**KEY USES**
- *Prevents infection in wounds.*
- *Stings, cuts, and grazes.*
- *Eye injuries.*
- *Rheumatic pain, where affected area feels cold.*

*Fresh plant is gathered when in flower in summer*

**WILD ROSEMARY △▷**
*This plant has antiseptic qualities. All parts are gathered, then dried and powdered to make the homeopathic remedy.*

# 39 LYCOPODIUM / CLUB MOSS

(*Lycopodium clavatum*) This is a well-known remedy for digestive complaints, particularly indigestion. In men, it can increase libido for those with an inability to achieve a sustained erection. Ailments tend to be right-sided, with a desire for sweet foods. Symptoms are better for loosening the clothes and for movement, and worse for overeating.

**KEY USES**
- *Digestive disorders.*
- *Enlarged prostate.*
- *Kidney and bladder problems.*
- *Right-sided complaints.*
- *Emotional problems due to insecurity.*

*Flowering spikes collected*

*Tiny spores and powder shaken out*

△ **CLUB MOSS**
*The remedy is made from the spores and yellow pollen dust shaken from the spikes.*

# 40 NUX VOMICA / POISON NUT

(*Strychnos nux vomica*) This remedy is mainly given for extreme over-sensitivity and irritability. People needing the remedy feel angry and frustrated when their expectations are not met, and become ill and feel stressed when they bottle up their anger. Digestive complaints, such as indigestion, vomiting, diarrhoea with painful cramps, nausea, and constipation, brought on through the suppression of emotions or over-indulgence in certain foods or stimulants, all benefit from this remedy. Colds, flu, and retching or dry coughs, headaches, and migraines are also eased.

LEAVES ▷
*These also contain the poison, which has long been used in small doses to stimulate the appetite and aid the digestion.*

*Button-like seeds found in pulp of hard-shelled fruit*

POISON NUT ▷
*The leaves, bark, and seeds of this tree all contain strychnine, but the homeopathic remedy is made from the seeds.*

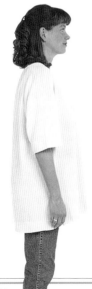

◁ FEMALE COMPLAINTS
*In women, Nux vomica is administered for labour pains. It is also given for morning sickness, cramps, and frequent urination in pregnancy; and for early, heavy, or irregular menstruation, and cystitis.*

KEY USES
• Digestive complaints.
• Insomnia and irritability caused by suppressing anger.
• Colds, flu with fever, and coughs also benefit.
• Headaches and migraines.
• Women's complaints.

# 41 PULSATILLA / PASQUE FLOWER

*(Pulsatilla pratensis) Pulsatilla* remedies treat conditions that are accompanied by a profuse yellow or yellowish-green discharge. These include colds with a runny or blocked nose, sinusitis, and loose coughs. Eye problems such as styes and conjunctivitis, and digestive complaints caused by rich foods, such as indigestion, gastroenteritis, nausea, and vomiting also benefit. *Pulsatilla* is an effective remedy for women's complaints, particularly those menstrual and menopausal problems that are characterized by weepiness, depression, and a need for comfort and concern. All symptoms are generally better for fresh air, gentle exercise, and crying and sympathy.

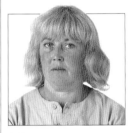

△ DEPRESSION
This remedy benefits depression characterized by weepiness and a lack of self-esteem and will-power, especially when it relates to women's menstrual and menopausal problems.

PASQUE FLOWER ▷
*The whole of the fresh plant, native to Russia, Germany, and Scandinavia, is pulped and the juice expressed is used to make the remedy.*

*Plant must be in flower when collected for remedy*

*The roots are also pulped to extract juice*

KEY USES
• *Ailments accompanied by a profuse yellowish-green discharge such as catarrh or conjunctivitis.*
• *Digestive problems caused by rich, fatty foods.*
• *Women's menstrual and menopausal complaints, often characterized by depression.*

# 42 RHUS TOX. / POISON IVY

(*Rhus toxicodendron*) *Rhus tox.* is mainly used to treat burning, itchy skin complaints that tend to scale like herpes, nappy rash, and eczema; and musculo-skeletal problems such as osteoarthritis, rheumatism, cramps, sprains, and strains. People needing this remedy may be anxious, irritable, and very sensitive to cold.

◁ POISON IVY
*Fresh leaves, which cause a violent skin rash, are collected before the plant flowers, and pounded to a pulp to make the remedy.*

KEY USES
• *Skin complaints where the skin is itchy, red, swollen, and burning.*
• *Joint and muscle ailments where stiffness and pain are better for continued movement, but worse on first starting to move.*
• *Heavy, prolonged, early menstruation.*
• *Symptoms of rheumatic fever and flu.*

# 43 RUTA GRAV. / RUE

(*Ruta Graveolens*) This is an important remedy for bruising of the lining of the bones which gives deep aching pain, rheumatism, tendon injuries, painful bruises, and sciatica. *Ruta grav.* is also given for eyestrain, with hot, red-looking eyes and eyestrain-induced headaches, often from reading very small print. Chest weakness and breathing difficulties, with pain over the breastbone, benefit as well. Symptoms are usually better for movement and worse for rest.

KEY USES
• *Bruised, aching bones and muscles.*
• *Eyestrain from fine, detailed work.*

RUE ▷
*The remedy is made from the whole fresh plant before it flowers. Sap may irritate.*

# 44 THUJA / WHITE CEDAR

*(Thuja occidentalis)* As well as being a key remedy for warts and genito-urinary tract conditions, physical symptoms that *Thuja* is given for include: offensive-smelling perspiration; stress-, excitement-, or exhaustion-induced headaches; tooth decay and swollen gums; and chronic catarrh. People who need this remedy are very sensitive and tend not to sleep well.

**KEY USES**
- *Warts and other skin complaints like oily skin.*
- *Nail problems.*
- *Remedy acts on the genito-urinary tract.*
- *Ailments characterized by yellowish-green or green catarrh.*
- *Menstrual problems.*

**WHITE CEDAR ▷**
*The aromatic leaves and twigs are pounded to a pulp to make the homeopathic remedy. A cream from the pulp helps rheumatism.*

# 45 URTICA / STINGING NETTLE

*(Urtica urens)* This remedy can be taken either internally or applied externally as an ointment, and is mainly given for skin problems, often due to an allergic reaction. Burns, where the skin is hot and blistered, and eczema, when the skin is itchy or blotchy, are both helped by *Urtica*. It is effective for rheumatism and is given for acute gout, nerve inflammation, and neuralgia.

**◁ STINGING NETTLE**
*The whole fresh plant of this common worldwide weed is used to make the remedy. The plant is covered in soft hairs, which cause itching and inflammation on contact.*

**KEY USES**
- *Burning and stinging skin complaints.*
- *Rheumatic pain.*
- *Burns with itching and swelling.*
- *Insect stings.*
- *Burning urine.*

# MINERAL REMEDIES

## 46 ARGENT. NIT. / SILVER NITRATE

*(Argentium nitricum)*

This remedy is used for fear and anxiety brought on by an over-active imagination. It is given for digestive complaints precipitated by nervous excitement or eating too many sweet foods. *Argent. nit.* is effective for pain that is better for pressure and fresh air, but worse for movement or talking. Complaints are usually left-sided.

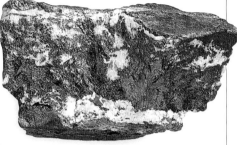

△ ACANTHITE
*This mineral is found in Norway, the USA, and South America. It is the main ore of silver.*

SILVER NITRATE ▷
*The homeopathic remedy is made from silver nitrate, which is extracted from the mineral acanthite. It is mainly used for nervous and digestive problems.*

*Crystals of silver nitrate*

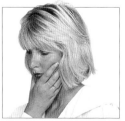

ANXIETIES & FEARS
*This remedy helps stage-fright, claustrophobia, and anxiety in the face of unexpected situations.*

KEY USES
- *Anxieties, fears, and phobias.*
- *Digestive complaints brought about through nervous excitement.*
- *Ailments that are accompanied by a craving for sweet foods.*

# 47 ARSEN. ALB. / ARSENIC

*(Arsenicum album)* Arsen. alb. is given for anxiety that is caused by underlying insecurity and over-sensitivity. This remedy is effective for a range of digestive disorders. Among these are: food poisoning, indigestion, diarrhoea, and gastroenteritis from too many ripe fruit and vegetables, from iced foods, or from drinking too much alcohol. The remedy is given for fevers where the person is hot to the touch but feels cold inside, or cold to the touch but feels very hot inside.

KEY USES
• *Anxiety and fear due to deep-seated insecurity.*
• *Digestive disorders and mucous membranes that are inflamed, especially in the digestive tract.*
• *Ailments with burning pain, better for heat.*

*Crystals have metallic lustre*

◁ ARSENOPHRYTE
*This mineral is the main ore of arsenic. When the crystals are heated they give off a smell of garlic. The remedy is made from arsenic oxide.*

# 48 AURUM MET. / GOLD

*(Aurum metallicum)* People who need this remedy are very sensitive to being contradicted. It is used for mental illnesses, such as depression. Increased circulation that causes congestion of blood in the head and other organs; heart disease; liver problems; sinusitis; and bone pain to do with bone loss also benefit from *Aurum met.*

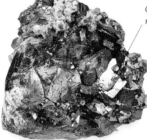

△ GOLD
*This dense, precious metal is still used in orthodox medicine and dentistry.*

KEY USES
• *Depression and suicidal thoughts related to fear of failure.*
• *Congestion of blood associated with vascular complaints.*
• *Ailments characterized by general over-sensitivity to noise, smell, touch, taste, and music.*

GOLD POWDER ▷
*Pure gold is ground down to a fine powder to make the homeopathic remedy.*

*Fine powder*

# 49 CALC. CARB.

(*Calcarea carbonica*) This remedy is mainly used to treat slow development of bones and teeth; joint and bone pain such as backache; slow-to-heal fractures; and painful teething in children. Ear infections with a sour-smelling discharge, and eye infections, where the white of the eye is red, are treated with *Calc. carb.* Other conditions helped by it include: eczema; thrush; PMS; heavy menstruation; menopausal symptoms; and digestive disorders.

*Important middle layer*

△ OYSTER SHELL
*The mother-of-pearl layer contains calcium carbonate, which is made into the remedy.*

*Sharp tool scrapes out mother-of-pearl*

OYSTER SHELL POWDER ▷
*The middle layer of the oyster shell is ground to a powder to make the homeopathic remedy.*

*Contains calcium carbonate*

*Shell is dried thoroughly, then powdered*

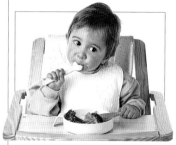

PAINFUL TEETHING
Calc. carb. *has many wide-ranging applications but acts on the bones and teeth in particular. It is therefore good for a child experiencing painful teething, with sore gums, sweaty scalp, and fever.*

KEY USES
• *Slow development of bones and teeth.*
• *Joint and bone pain.*
• *Ailments characterized by fears and anxieties, profuse, sour-smelling perspiration, and sensitivity to cold.*
• *Right-sided headaches.*
• *Women's complaints, such as heavy menstruation and menopausal symptoms.*

# 50 CALC. PHOS. / CALCIUM PHOSPHATE

(*Calcarea phosphorica*) The *Calc. phos.* remedy is mainly used to treat bone complaints, such as painful bones and joints or slow-to-heal fractures, and rapid tooth decay. It is also good for problems such as slow growth and growing pain in children. It helps weakness and fatigue after illness, and is a key remedy for digestive disorders. In children, *Calc. phos.* is effective for delayed teething. Glue ear and recurrent tonsillitis are prevalent in children who need this remedy.

KEY USES
• *Pain in bones and teeth.*
• *Problems associated with growth in children and adolescents.*
• *Mental and physical weakness.*
• *Digestive problems.*
• *Discontented feelings.*

▽ BONES
*Calcium phosphate (formed by a chemical reaction to make the remedy) is a constituent of bones.*

*Calcium phosphate makes bones hard*

# 51 CARBO VEG. / CHARCOAL

(*Carbo vegitibilis*) This remedy is mainly given for exhaustion, weakness, and low vitality following an operation or illness. It is also given for lack of oxygenation in the tissues due to poor venous circulation. Symptoms include cold, bluish skin on the hands, feet, and face; and puffy, cold legs. Digestive problems, regardless of diet, are helped by this remedy, as are asthma and spasmodic coughing.

KEY USES
• *Low vitality and exhaustion.*
• *Cold, clammy skin but feeling hot inside, associated with shock.*
• *Conditions affecting venous circulation and digestion.*

*Charcoal is a form of carbon*

◁ △ CARBO VEG. REMEDY
*This remedy comes from charcoal, which is made from partly burnt wood. It helps people suffering from exhaustion to feel more vital.*

39

# 52 CUPRUM MET. / COPPER

(*Cuprum metallicum*) This remedy mainly affects the nervous system and is used to treat cramps that start in the toes and spread into the feet, ankles, and calves. It is effective for the convulsions and muscular spasms of epilepsy. *Cuprum met.* is good for respiratory problems such as asthma and whooping cough, when breathing can seem to stop.

**COPPER** △ ▷
*This reddish-gold metal was the first to be used to make tools and weapons. It is powdered for the homeopathic remedy.*

KEY USES
• *Cramps in the feet, ankles, and calves*
• *Epilepsy, with muscular spasms that start in the fingers and toes and move in.*
• *Tiredness or exhaustion from mental exertion.*
• *Respiratory problems.*

# 53 FERRUM PHOS. / IRON

(*Ferrum phosphoricum*) Ferrum phos. is used for the onset of infections and inflammations, such as slow-starting fevers and dry, hacking coughs with chest pain; colds that start slowly; laryngitis; headaches eased by cool compresses; earache; indigestion; rheumatism with a temperature and shooting pain; and the early stages of dysentery. People needing this remedy dislike meat and milk, and crave caffeine.

**VIVIANITE** ▽
*This mineral is a natural source of iron phosphate, from which the remedy is made. It is usually prepared chemically.*

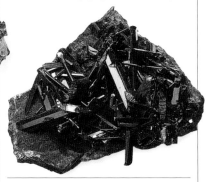

KEY USES
• *The early stages of inflammation, fever, and infection before any other definite symptoms have appeared.*
• *Coughs and colds that are slow to start, and may start with a nosebleed.*
• *A weak and rapid pulse rate.*

# 54 GRAPHITES / GRAPHITE

*(Graphites)* This is a key remedy for skin complaints, especially weeping eczema with a honey-like discharge, often behind the ears and the knees, on the palms of the hands, and on the nipples. It is also good for people with a metabolic imbalance that may cause skin complaints such as psoriasis and dry, cracked skin; cuts that become septic; scar tissue that hardens; and thick, cracked, and misshapen nails. Symptoms are better for warmth, for sleep, and for eating.

**KEY USES**
• *Skin complaints, especially eczema.*
• *Metabolic imbalances that lead to skin problems and obesity.*
• *Ulcers caused by a weakness in the stomach lining.*

GRAPHITE △▷
*This mineral occurs in older crystalline rocks, marble, and granite. Graphite is ground to a powder to make the homeopathic remedy.*

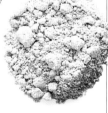

# 55 HEPAR SULPH. / CALCIUM SULPHIDE

*(Hepar sulphuris calcareum)* Hepar sulph. is mainly used for infections sensitive to touch, for example in tonsillitis, earache, and some skin problems; and helps to expel pus in infected spots or boils. It is also given for sore throats with ear pain on swallowing; sinusitis; coughs; and flu with a fever, sneezing, sweating, and a need for warmth. The secretions of people treated with this remedy when ill often smell sour.

**KEY USES**
• *Infection, especially with the formation of pus.*
• *Ailments characterized by sharp pain, sour-smelling secretions and sensitivity to touch.*
• *Sore throat with ear pain.*

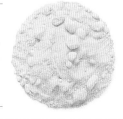

△ OYSTER SHELL
*The inside layer of an oyster shell is ground to a powder before mixing.*

◁ FLOWERS OF SULPHUR
*This is mixed with oyster shell powder, and heated to make the remedy.*

# 56 KALI BICH. / POTASSIUM DICHROMATE

*(Kali bichromicum)* This remedy eases complaints affecting the mucous membranes, especially in the nose, throat, vagina, urethra, and stomach. It is an important remedy for catarrhal conditions, such as colds that turn into sinusitis. *Kali bich.* is used to treat joint problems with rheumatic pain that appears and disappears suddenly. Digestive disorders, such as nausea and vomiting of yellow mucus; and migraines that start at night also benefit from this remedy. Symptoms are better for heat and movement.

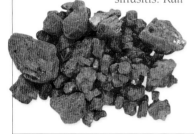

◁ **KALI BICH.**
*This remedy is chemically prepared from the bright orange particles of pure potassium dichromate.*

**KEY USES**
• *Thick, stringy, yellow or white mucus and other forms of discharge.*
• *Pain that shifts rapidly about the body, and often appears and disappears.*

# 57 KALI PHOS. / POTASSIUM PHOSPHATE

*(Kali phosphoricum)* People experiencing mental and physical exhaustion, with nervousness and over-sensitivity caused by extreme stress or over-exertion, benefit most from this remedy. Physical symptoms of this exhaustion include: sensitivity to cold; a yellow-coated tongue; a yellow or pus-filled discharge; and extreme muscular weakness. Their symptoms are better for eating.

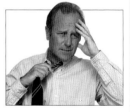

**SYMPTOMS OF STRESS**
*People who need this remedy tend to sweat on the face and head from excitement or after meals.*

◁ **POTASSIUM PHOSPHATE**
*The remedy is prepared chemically by adding phosphoric acid to a solution of potassium carbonate.*

**KEY USES**
• *Physical and mental exhaustion with an associated aversion to company and marked chilliness.*
• *Pus-filled discharges.*

# 58 MERC. SOL. / MERCURY

*(Hydragyrum metallicum)* Merc. sol. is effective for a wide range of conditions accompanied by profuse, burning, smelly secretions, and an associated sensitivity to heat and cold. It is used for mouth and throat complaints with a thirst for cold drinks. *Merc. sol.* is also a good remedy for eye complaints; nasal problems due to a cold or allergy; and skin conditions with blisters and ulcers.

### KEY USES
• *Ailments accompanied by profuse, strong-smelling, burning bodily discharges; sensitivity to heat and cold.*
• *Ailments of the throat and mouth, such as tonsillitis.*

◁△ MERCURY
*This is often found in the mineral cinnabar (above). Liquid mercury is then dissolved in dilute nitric acid. The precipitate that results is powdered (left) to make the remedy.*

# 59 NATRUM MUR. / ROCK SALT

*(Natrum muriaticum)* Homeopaths give this remedy for emotional problems that are caused by suppressed grief and other emotions. *Natrum mur.* is also used to treat conditions with a watery discharge, such as colds and catarrh with a profuse, clear mucus. Complaints that are often brought on by stuffy heat or exposure to hot sun, such as migraines, headaches, and cold sores, also benefit.

▽ ROCK SALT
*Also known as sodium chloride, rock salt is formed when saline water evaporates. This is then used to make the remedy.*

### KEY USES
• *Emotional problems caused by suppressed feelings, especially grief.*
• *Ailments accompanied by discharges that look like the white of an egg.*
• *Complaints that are worse for heat.*

# 60 PHOS. / PHOSPHORUS

(*Phosphorus*) This remedy is given for anxieties and fears that cause nervous tension, insomnia, and exhaustion. It treats circulatory problems; profuse bleeding in the form of nosebleeds, bleeding gums, heavy menstrual flow, and bleeding from the stomach lining are also all eased by *Phos*. Digestive complaints and some respiratory problems (asthma, bronchitis, and pneumonia) are alleviated.

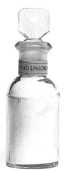

*Phosphorus is highly flammable*

## KEY USES
- *Anxieties and fears.*
- *Problems of bleeding and circulation.*
- *Digestive disorders.*
- *Respiratory complaints.*
- *Ailments characterized by burning pain.*

◁△ PHOSPHORUS
*This mineral, from which the remedy is made, is one of the most important for life. It is found in our bones and body fluids.*

# 61 SILICEA / ROCK CRYSTAL

(*Silicea terra*) *Silicea* is mainly used for undernourishment that leads to a weakened immune system and recurrent infections, such as colds, flu, and ear infections. It is effective for skin and bone complaints: spotty complexion; weak nails; slow-to-heal fractures; and fontanelles that are slow to close. Nervous system problems also benefit.

▽△ SILICA
*This is the main constituent of most rocks such as flint (above) and rock crystal (left). To make the homeopathic remedy, however, silica is usually prepared chemically.*

## KEY USES
- *Recurrent infections caused by general under-nourishment.*
- *Skin and bone problems.*
- *Expelling splinters and other foreign bodies.*
- *Problems of the nerves.*

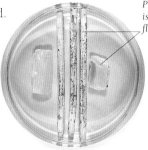

# 62 SULPHUR

(*Sulphur*) Skin conditions, such as eczema, thrush, or nappy rash where the skin appears permanently dirty and is dry, scaly, itchy, hot, red, and worse for scratching, all benefit from Sulphur, as does dry scalp. Digestive complaints that are helped by this remedy include a tendency to regurgitate food; indigestion worsened by drinking milk; vomiting and chronic diarrhoea; and piles and itching around the anus. In women, it benefits the symptoms of both PMS and menopause.

**FLOWERS OF SULPHUR ▷**
*Lumps of fine yellow powder are extracted from mineral sulphur. When burnt, flowers of sulphur gives off sulphur dioxide, which is a powerful disinfectant.*

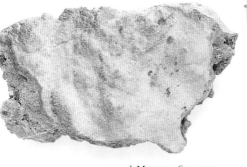

△ **GROUND TO POWDER**
*Flowers of sulphur is ground to a powder that is soluble in alcohol to make the homeopathic remedy.*

△ **MINERAL SULPHUR**
*This is to be found near volcanic craters and hot springs in Italy and the USA.*

**KEY USES**
• *Skin conditions, mostly eczema, where the skin is inflamed, itchy, and hot.*
• *Digestive disorders.*
• *Women's complaints.*
• *Mental stresses such as lack of energy and will power, forgetfulness, irritability and indecision.*

**DRY SCALP ▷**
*One of the skin conditions that Sulphur benefits is a scalp that is dry and itchy. Scratching the scalp will make the itching worse.*

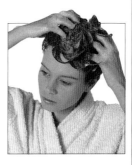

# USING THE REMEDIES

## 63 ESSENTIAL GUIDELINES

While it is always wise to seek the help of medical practitioners or homeopaths for chronic, long-term conditions, or if your symptoms worsen, many common complaints can be treated at home, using homeopathic remedies available from chemists and health shops. Because the remedies have been diluted repeatedly, they are safe and there are no long-term side-effects. Try to match your symptoms as closely as possible to the remedy information.

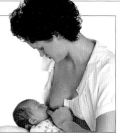

**LACTATING MOTHERS**
*Mothers can take homeopathic remedies while breast-feeding, and they are safe for babies. Try to avoid them during pregnancy, but consult a homeopath to be sure.*

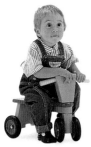

◁ **SAFE FOR CHILDREN?**
*Because the remedies are so diluted, they are very safe for children, even if several tablets are inadvertently swallowed.*

**AGE LIMIT?** ▷
*Homeopathic remedies are just as safe for the elderly as anyone else, provided their symptoms are always matched as closely as possible to the remedy.*

**CONSULTING A HOMEOPATH**
• *If you have doubts about treating yourself, consult a homeopath for advice first.*
• *Consult a homeopath for recurrent ailments.*
• *If symptoms worsen for more than a few hours, seek professional help.*
• *If symptoms do not improve within the recommended time of taking the remedy, consult a professional.*

# 64 STORING HOMEOPATHIC REMEDIES

Remedies should be stored in a cool, dark place, well away from food or other products with a strong smell. It is best to use dark glass bottles, and always make sure that the tops of the containers are screwed on tightly. If stored properly, remedies will last for many years. As with all medicines, keep out of reach of children, although the remedies will not cause more than transient diarrhoea if taken in excess.

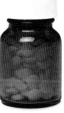

DARK GLASS BOTTLE

# 65 GETTING THE MOST FROM YOUR REMEDY

It is best not to take more than one remedy at a time. Do not touch the remedy: drop it onto your tongue from a clean, dry spoon, and do not take with food or drink: wait 30 minutes. Avoid wearing perfume and using strong-smelling household cleaners. Some essential oils have an antidoting effect.

◁ MINT LEAF

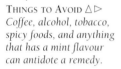

THINGS TO AVOID △▷
*Coffee, alcohol, tobacco, spicy foods, and anything that has a mint flavour can antidote a remedy.*

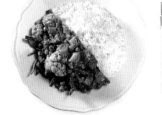

# 66 TAKING THE CORRECT DOSE

Homeopathic remedies, like orthodox medicines, should be taken when needed and stopped as soon as possible. If your symptoms become worse, it may be a sign that the remedy is working, but this worsening should only last for a few hours and then you should begin to feel better. If this happens, stop taking the remedy and let your immune system take over. If there is no improvement, consult a professional.

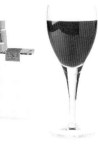

LACTOSE TABLETS

# MINOR AILMENTS

## 67 MUSCULAR PAIN

Rheumatism is the general term for muscular aches and pains. Symptoms may be caused by viral infection or food allergy, or there may be an underlying joint disease. The pain may be constant or vary in intensity according to the weather or hormonal changes. Cramp is caused by a spasm in the muscles due to a lack of oxygen and build-up of waste products. Acute pain in the muscles may be due to an injury that damages the muscle fibres, tendons, and ligaments, and causes stiffness, swelling, and loss of movement. Consult a doctor following all but minor injuries.

Orthodox medicine has not yet identified the causes for restless legs. They are often due to problems with the nervous system, and most sufferers have an iron deficiency.

CRAMP IN FOOT OR LEG ▷
*Cramp or muscle spasm can be caused by fatigue from too much exercise, or by loss of body salt through sweating or vomiting.*

SEEK MEDICAL ADVICE
• *If muscle pain (and bone or joint pain) becomes severe and persistent, consult a doctor within 12 hours.*
• *Even if there is no deterioration, if the pain had not responded to the appropriate homeopathic remedy in 14 days, seek medical advice.*
• *Improving diet and taking nutritional supplements can help muscular aches and pains in the long term.*

| AILMENT | SYMPTOMS | REMEDY | |
|---|---|---|---|
| Severe cramp in the feet or legs | Starts with a twitching of the muscles, leading to violent muscle spasms. | *Bryonia* see p.25 | |
| Cramp from muscle fatigue | Bruised cramping pain after over-exertion; limbs feel as if they have been beaten. | *Cuprum met.* see p.40 | |
| Restless legs | Restlessness; tickling feeling like ants under the skin; burning prickling sensations. | *Rhus tox.* see p.34 | |

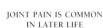

# 68 Joint & bone pain

Flu is a common cause of bone pain, while inactivity, bad posture, poor working position, or an underlying emotional problem can all cause joint and muscle pain. Osteoarthritis is cause by the wearing away of the cartilage that lines the joints as a result of age, obesity, injury, or overuse. It results in limited movement, pain, and occasionally acute inflammation. Many people over 40 suffer to some degree, often in the weight-bearing joints. As well as the treatments below, nutritional and herbal supplements may help.

JOINT PAIN IS COMMON IN LATER LIFE

| Ailment | Symptoms | Remedy |
|---------|----------|--------|
| Pain with stiffness | Restlessness and irritability; stiffness and aching pain in affected joints on waking. | Rhus tox. see p.34 |
| Severe pain on movement | Hot, swollen joints that are excruciatingly painful with the slightest movement. | Bryonia see p.25 |
| Pain accompanied by weeping | Emotional and tearful; pain flits from one joint to another; desire for sympathy. | Pulsatilla see p.33 |
| Pain aggravated by injury | Bruising pain, sore to touch; movement difficult; system in shock; desire to be alone. | Arnica see p.24 |
| Pain brought on by movement | Aches and pains worse for moving, better for rest; pain is associated with dull feeling. | Bryonia see p.25 |
| Rheumatic pain with weepiness | Pain flits from one joint to another; desire for sympathy and consolation. | Pulsatilla see p.33 |
| Pain eased by prolonged gentle movement | Aching stiffness worse on waking; worsens then eases on moving; restlessness. | Rhus tox. see p.34 |
| Stiffness due to contracted tendons | Pain with muscle spasms in jaw and neck; stiff neck in a draught; tearing muscle pain. | Causticum Ask your homeopath for details of this remedy. |
| Pain in the tendons | Pain appears after tendon injuries, or where bone lining had become bruised and sore. | Ruta grav. see p.34 |

# 69 HEADACHES & MIGRAINES

Unless caused by injury, homeopaths view headaches and migraines as symptomatic of an imbalance in the body. Most headaches are due to muscular tension, rheumatism in the neck, sinusitis, or PMS. Migraines are severe headaches and may be hormonal.

| AILMENT | SYMPTOMS | REMEDY | |
|---------|----------|--------|---|
| Violent headache that comes on suddenly | Sudden severe pain; brain feels too big; feeling of tight band around head; anxiety. | *Aconite* see p.22 | |
| Throbbing headache from heat | Throbbing, drumming headache; face becomes red, pupils enlarged; delirium. | *Belladonna* see p.25 | |
| Bursting, crushing headache | Stabbing pain from eye movement; head feels as if it will break; no desire to talk. | *Bryonia* see p.25 | |
| Headache caused by emotional stress | Very severe pain; sensation of a tight band across forehead, or a nail in the side of head. | *Ignatia* see p.30 | |
| Headache from muscular tension in the neck | Feeling of pressure at top of head, or a full sensation; eye pain; neck stiffness or spasms. | *Cimic.* see p.26 | |
| Headache from a hangover, with nausea | Sensation of weight bearing down on head; dizziness; tendency to be hypercritical. | *Nux vomica* see p.32 | |
| Blinding, throbbing migraine | Begins with numbness and tingling in lips and tongue; severe pulsating pain. | *Natrum mur.* see p.43 | |
| Migraine accompanied by weepiness | Associated with moodiness and changeable emotions; head feels it will burst; crying. | *Pulsatilla* see p.33 | |

# 70 HANGOVER CURES

When you have a hangover from drinking alcohol, try to sleep, keep warm, and apply pressure to the affected part of your head. Washing your hair may be soothing. Avoid noise, more alcohol, being touched, and if possible, cold winds.

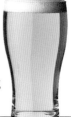

◁ DRINKING
*Prevention is always better than cure, so if possible pace yourself when drinking, and drink plenty of water.*

# 71 TEETH, MOUTH, & GUMS

Although they are common, problems with teeth, mouth, and gums can be prevented with good oral hygiene, regular check-ups, and eating fibrous, non-sugary foods. If there is fever and swelling of the face, or a tooth feels loose, see a dentist as soon as possible.

| AILMENT | SYMPTOMS | REMEDY |
|---|---|---|
| Toothache with throbbing pain | Gums and cheeks are hot, sore, and swollen; pain first increases then subsides. | *Belladonna* *see p.25* |
| Bleeding gums and bad breath | Tender, spongy gums that bleed easily; excessive saliva; teeth may feel loose. | *Merc. sol.* *see p.43* |
| Swollen, bleeding gums with ulcers | Taste of pus; teeth sensitive to heat and cold; possible mouth ulcers and cold sores. | *Natrum mur.* *see p.43* |
| Burning mouth ulcers | Mouth feels dry; smarting pain; restlessness and anxiety. | *Arsen. alb.* *see p.37* |
| Cold sores on the lips and around the mouth | Mouth feels dry; lips swollen with blisters; cracked lower lip; desire to be left alone. | *Natrum. mur.* *see p.43* |
| Bad breath caused by tooth decay or inflamed gums | Breath and sweat smell offensive; excessive saliva; tongue yellow and coated. | *Merc. sol.* *see p.43* |
| Immediate discomfort after dental treatment | Discomfort after any dental work, especially where there has been trauma and bruising. | *Arnica* *see p.24* |
| Persistent pain after dental treatment | Pain continues after initial discomfort, or returns once the anaesthetic has worn off. | *Hypericum* *see p.29* |

# 72 EARACHE

All earaches, but particularly in children, should be referred promptly to a doctor. They can be caused by a build-up of wax, or an infection in the outer, middle, or inner ear, after a cold for example. Temperature extremes make it hard for the body's healing powers to fight infection. Until you see a doctor, take *Hepar sulph.* (see p.41) for sharp pain, and *Belladonna* (see p.25) for throbbing pain.

# 73 EYE COMPLAINTS

Eyestrain can be caused by overwork or working in poor light. Stress, especially after an emotional upset or resulting from grief, can weaken eye muscles and cause eyestrain.

Conjunctivitis or swelling of the eyelid lining is caused by an infection or allergy, and will feel worse for being indoors, in warmth, and in light. Styes are small pus-filled boils that form at the base of the eyelashes, caused by infection and aggravated by tiredness. Anything that weakens the immune system's ability to fight infection, like temperature extremes, fatigue, and stress, can aggravate eye conditions.

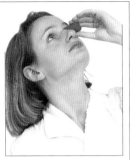

**HOMEOPATHIC EYE BATH**
*Add two drops of Euphrasia mother tincture to an eyebath of cooled, salted water for a soothing rinse.*

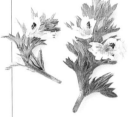

◁ **EYEBRIGHT**
*This small wildflower, used to make the remedy Euphrasia, was first mentioned in the 14th century as a medicine for eyes.*

**PRECAUTIONS**
*Always consult a doctor if:*
• *there is no improvement in conjunctivitis in 24 hours*
• *there is no improvement in styes within seven days.*

| AILMENT | SYMPTOMS | REMEDY |
|---|---|---|
| Eyes ache on movement | Dull, aching pain on looking up, down, or sideways; dislike of sympathy. | *Natrum mur.* see p.43 |
| Burning eyes | Eyes burn and feel strained after prolonged reading; eyes are red and hot; headache. | *Ruta grav.* see p.34 |
| Swollen eyelids with a burning discharge | Eyes water continuously; need to blink frequently; little blisters inside eyelids. | *Euphrasia* see p.28 |
| Swollen eyes with itchy eyelids | Eyes red and inflamed; small boils with head of pus; may feel depressed. | *Pulsatilla* see p.33 |
| Swollen, red painful eyes | Styes start as small boils at base of the eyelashes, and then develop a head of pus. | *Staphysagria* Ask your homeopath for details of this remedy. |

# 74 HAY FEVER & ALLERGIES

Like the ears and eyes, the nose is continually assaulted by dust particles, spores, chemicals, viruses, bacteria, smoke, and pollution, all of which can cause problems. Hay fever, or allergic rhinitis is a seasonal allergic reaction to air-borne irritants – usually pollen. If it continues throughout the year, it is usually due to animal fur or house dust. If you suffer from allergies try to include plenty of fresh raw fruits and vegetables in your daily diet, and take magnesium and vitamin C supplements, as a deficiency of essential vitamins and minerals may lead to increased sensitivity.

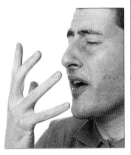

**DESIRE TO SNEEZE**
*Certain types of hay fever are characterized by violent sneezing. Sadly, it usually brings no relief.*

| AILMENT | SYMPTOMS | REMEDY |
|---|---|---|
| Hay fever with a burning nasal discharge | Streaming, burning nasal discharge; pain in forehead; larynx scratchy; eyes stream. | *Allium* see p.23 |
| Hay fever with a constant desire to sneeze | Thick nasal discharge after 3–4 days of violent sneezing; sore nostrils; burning throat. | *Arsen iod.* Ask your homeopath for details of this remedy. |
| Hay fever where the eyes are mainly affected | Eyes swollen and sensitive; thick burning discharge from eyes; post-nasal drip. | *Euphrasia* see p.28 |
| Hay fever with a sore throat | Sore throat, often starting on left side; sore to swallow; dry throat; eyes water; sneezing. | *Sabadilla* Ask your homeopath for details of this remedy. |

# 75 HAIR LOSS

Loss of hair is common in both men and women as they get older, although baldness is hereditary and occurs mainly in men. Hair loss can also be caused by fever, childbirth, shock, stress or an excess or lack of vitamin A and selenium (both of which are found in vegetables, fish, and eggs). If there is unexplained, sudden hair loss, it is wise to see a doctor. If you experience premature balding or greying because of childbirth or premature ageing, take *Lycopodium*, (*see p.31*). Take 6c every 12 hours for up to one month.

# 76 SKIN COMPLAINTS

Homeopaths view skin complaints as a reflection of overall health, rather than just a local condition. Stress or poor nutrition can manifest in a skin problem, although allergy and infection may also be responsible. Lack of exercise, constipation, sugar, spices, caffeine, and alcohol are the main aggravating factors.

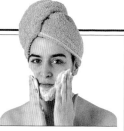

**ACNE ACTION**
*Never squeeze or pick acne; wash very carefully.*

| AILMENT | SYMPTOMS | REMEDY |
|---------|----------|--------|
| Moist eczema with a honey-like discharge | Rough, dry, or cracked skin, mainly palms and behind ears; skin may turn septic. | *Graphites* see p.41 |
| Dry eczema | Dry, rough, red, itchy skin; associated with diarrhoea, wrong foods, and alcohol. | *Sulphur* see p.45 |
| Moist eczema with skin that cracks easily | Sensitive, rough, broken skin; scratches become pus-filled, cracked and bleed; crusts itch. | *Petroleum* Ask your homeopath for details of this remedy. |
| Itchy pimples on the face, chest, and shoulders | Blackheads; pustules with depressed centre; associated with excess sexual urges. | *Kali brom.* Ask your homeopath for details of this remedy. |
| Large, painful, pus-filled spots | Spots are extremely painful to touch; blackheads worse on forehead. | *Hepar sulph.* see p.41 |
| Spots associated with a hormonal imbalance | Spots worse at puberty as menstruation begins; mainly in those who are overweight. | *Pulsatilla* see p.33 |
| Swelling, mostly on the lips and eyelids | Red, swollen, burning skin; possible depression and sensitivity; throat swelling. | *Apis, see p.18* See a doctor if throat swells. |
| Urticaria (hives) with violently itchy blotches | Burning sensation on hands and fingers; itchy, red, or pale slightly raised blotches. | *Urtica* see p.35 |
| Boils: early stages when the boil is starting to form | Affected skin is round and hard; swelling is painful, dry, burning, throbbing, and red. | *Belladonna* see p.25 |
| Boils: later stages, when pus has formed | Boil is sensitive to slightest touch, and is on the point of bursting. | *Hepar sulph.* see p.41 |

# 77 WOMEN'S HEALTH

Physical and emotional problems to do with the reproductive cycle are generally due to a hormone imbalance. Homeopaths also assess lifestyle factors to help restore balance. See a doctor if thrush does not clear up in five days; if menstruation changes at all; or if there is irregular bleeding in menopause.

**PREGNANCY PRECAUTIONS**
*Take homeopathic remedies during pregnancy only if necessary. Morning sickness, frequent urination, breast pain, heartburn, and labour pain can be helped, but see a homeopath for guidance.*

| AILMENT | SYMPTOMS | REMEDY | |
|---|---|---|---|
| Thrush with an itchy, milky discharge | Itching worse after urination and before menstruation; chronic headache, anxiety. | *Calc. carb.* see p.38 | |
| Thrush with a very offensive discharge | Vaginal and vulval itching; soreness and burning; ulcers; discharge worse after sex. | *Sepia* see p.21 | |
| Thrush with burning pain | Discharge causes itching; alternating diarrhoea and constipation; pain during sex. | *Sulphur* see p.45 | |
| PMS with fluid retention, swollen tender breasts | Painful joints; lack of energy; thrush; depression; loss of concentration; weepiness. | *Calc. carb.* see p.38 | |
| PMS with extreme weepiness | Depression, self-pity, tears for no reason; anxiety; desire for sweet foods; headaches. | *Pulsatilla* see p.33 | |
| Heavy menstruation, and weight gain | Bright red blood; cramps; irregular menstruation; anxiety; backache; clumsiness. | *Calc. carb.* see p.38 | |
| Heavy menstruation, faint and irritable | Severe cramps cause fainting; visual disturbance; itchy discharge; sweating; crying. | *Sepia.* see p.21 | |
| Painful menstrual cramps with marked weepiness | Severe pain can cause nausea and vomiting; tearing pain in lower abdomen; diarrhoea. | *Pulsatilla* see p.33 | |
| Menstruation stops suddenly | Aching pain in ovaries; sharp, shooting pain in uterus; fear, anxiety, and nervousness. | *Aconite* see p.22 | |
| Menopause with aversion to sexual intercourse | Vaginal pain during sex due to dryness; anxiety about sex; heavy, irregular menstruation. | *Sepia* see p.21 | |

# COUGHS & COLDS

## 78 COLDS & FLU

Both colds and flu are caused by a viral infection. They occur when the immune system is weakened, making the body susceptible to infections. This may be due to a poor diet; exposure to dry, cold, windy weather; becoming chilled after getting the head wet; insufficient rest; or emotional stress. Homeopathy emphasizes treating the underlying imbalance in the immune system, as well as fighting infection. If fever from flu does not clear within four days, see a doctor.

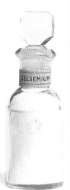

GELSEMIUM ▷
*This remedy is given for ailments with symptoms of fever, although the plant root from which it is made is toxic.*

| AILMENT | SYMPTOMS | REMEDY |
|---|---|---|
| Colds that come on slowly | Mouth feels hot; throat is red and swollen; mild fever; possible nosebleeds. | *Ferrum phos.* see p.40 |
| Cold with irritability | Chilliness; runny nose in the day, blocked at night; watery eyes; sneezing; headache. | *Nux vomica* see p.32 |
| Early stages of a cold with sneezing | Violent sneezing; nose blocked; desire to be alone; dislike of sympathy. | *Natrum mur.* see p.43 |
| Cold with yellow mucus | Nose blocked at night, but runny in the day; bland, yellow mucus; loss of smell. | *Pulsatilla* see p.33 |
| Flu with high fever | Sudden high fever; flushed, red face; sore throat; staring, wide eyes; possible delirium. | *Belladonna* see p.25 |
| Flu with chills and weakness | Lack of thirst despite fever; sore throat; chills; bursting headache; fatigue; bone pain. | *Gelsemium* see p.28 |
| Flu with severe throbbing headache | Violent headache, worse for coughing and moving eyes; dehydration; irritability. | *Bryonia* see p.25 |

# 79 CATARRH & SINUSITIS

Catarrh is a discharge of runny or sticky mucus, which may block the nose, resulting in pain. It can be caused by infection or allergy. Pollution irritates the mucous membranes causing more mucus in an attempt remove the irritation.

Sinusitis occurs if the sinuses become irritated or inflamed. They may fill with fluid, creating pressure and causing pain. This may be from pollution, smoke, or viral infection. If pain is very severe, see a doctor within 12 hours.

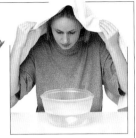

**SINUSITIS INHALATION**
*A steam inhalation can relieve the congestion in your sinuses, lessening the pressure, and easing pain.*

◁ **HYDRASTIS CANADENSIS**
*The remedy Hydrastis, made from the plant root, treats catarrh and sinusitis.*

| AILMENT | SYMPTOMS | REMEDY |
|---|---|---|
| Thick, white catarrhal mucus | Occurs once inflammation is down in a cold; discharge is through nose or down throat. | *Kali mur.* Ask your homeopath for details of this remedy. |
| Catarrhal mucus like the white of raw egg | Loss of smell and taste; excessive transparent, fluid mucus is extremely profuse. | *Natrum mur.* see p.43 |
| Catarrh with a constantly runny nose | Nose runs constantly; yellow, thin, burning discharge; post-nasal drip; small nose ulcers. | *Hydrastis* see above |
| Catarrh with high sensitivity to strong smells | Painful to blow nose due to crusts; possible nosebleeds; acute sense of smell. | *Graphites* see p.41 |
| Sinusitis with stringy mucus | Greenish-yellow stringy mucus; feeling of blockage; violent sneezing; loss of smell. | *Kali bich.* see p.42 |
| Sinusitis accompanied by weepiness | Pain above eyes or in right cheekbone; yellow mucus; stuffy nose; weepiness. | *Pulsatilla* see p.33 |
| Sinusitis with facial tenderness | Facial bones tender to even slight touch; excessive yellow mucus; sneezing; irritability. | *Hepar sulph.* see p.41 |

# 80 COUGHS

These are usually due to an irritation of the lining of the air passages, for example, by mucus dripping down the throat during a cold, smoking, or pollen in hay fever sufferers. To get rid of the irritation, the lungs build up a pressure of air, which is suddenly expelled. Coughs may be dry or productive (bringing up mucus). If they are accompanied by a high fever, difficulty in breathing, and/or severe chest pain, consult a doctor. If there is no improvement within one to two days after a sudden onset of coughing from inhaling dust or fumes, you should also see a doctor.

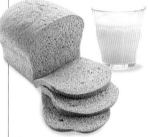

◁ **STARCHY FOODS & DAIRY PRODUCTS**
*If you are coughing up a lot of phlegm, avoid dairy products and starchy foods such as bread and potatoes, as these may cause the flow of mucus to increase.*

**THYME & LUNGWORT SYRUP** ▷
*Homeopathic and herbal cough syrups are available over the counter. They are preferable to orthodox syrups, which may cause drowsiness.*

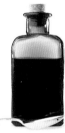

△ **LEMON & HONEY**
*Drink plenty of fluids when you have a cough. Hot water with lemon and honey is particularly beneficial.*

| AILMENT | SYMPTOMS | REMEDY | |
| --- | --- | --- | --- |
| Dry, irritating cough that comes on suddenly | Dry, hollow-sounding, croaking cough; great thirst; often a great temperature rise; anxiety; sensitivity to smoke. | *Aconite* see p.22 | |
| Chest pain from coughing | Bursting headache, worsened by even slight cough; extreme thirst; body feels dried out; may be accompanying fever. | *Bryonia* see p.25 | |
| Cough with thick green catarrh | Thick green mucus coughed up leaving bad taste in mouth; poor appetite; white-coated tongue; little thirst. | *Pulsatilla* see p.33 | |

# 81 THROAT COMPLAINTS

Throat disorders make breathing and swallowing difficult. They range from mild sore throats to more severe ailments such as tonsilitis and laryngitis. Common symptoms include a dry mouth and throat; inflammation causing a constricted sensation; hoarseness; bad breath; foul-tasting saliva; fatigue; and feeling feverish. Recurrent sore throats indicate a weakened immune system. If sore throats and tonsilitis are accompanied by fever, see a doctor.

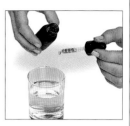

**SOOTHING THROAT GARGLE**
*Prepare a solution of five drops each of calendula and hypericum in water.*

| AILMENT | SYMPTOMS | REMEDY |
|---|---|---|
| Acute, painful sore throat | Sudden severe sore throat, causing anxiety; dry, hot skin; thirst; rough, burning throat. | *Aconite* see p.22 |
| Pain extends to the neck and ears | Bad taste; swallowing hurts; hot and cold by turns; heavy head; feel weary and weak. | *Gelsemium* see p.28 |
| Back of throat is bright red and severely swollen | Burning and stinging pain; back of throat is shiny, red, and swollen; seem irritable. | *Apis* see p.18 |
| Tonsillitis with burning pain that shoots into head | Sore throat; spasms of pain on moving; stiff, tender neck; red face; high fever. | *Belladonna* see p.25 |
| Tonsillitis with stabbing pain in throat | Throat feels as if a fish bone is stuck in it; bad breath; cough up pus; tend to shiver. | *Hepar sulph.* see p.41 |
| Tonsillitis with bad breath | Throat is dark red, sore, and swollen; swallowing hurts; yellow-coated swollen tongue. | *Merc. sol.* see p.43 |
| Laryngitis with a high fever | Hoarseness and loss of voice; sudden onset causes anxiety; appear restless. | *Aconite* see p.22 |
| Laryngitis with a dry, tickly cough | Dry, sore throat; hoarseness or loss of voice; talking is painful; thirst for cold drinks. | *Phos.* see p.44 |
| Loss of voice from too much singing or shouting | Tickly larynx; voice is weak, trembles and tends to break; hoarseness. | *Argent. nit.* see p.36 |

# EMOTIONAL PROBLEMS

## 82 ANXIETY & STRESS

These are very common and are caused by overwork, fear, or insecurity. They may manifest themselves physically in a fast pulse rate, clammy skin, and a disturbed appetite. If you have chest pain from severe anxiety, call an ambulance.

AVOID CAFFEINE ▷
*Cola drinks, tea, and coffee should all be avoided if you are feeling anxious.*

| Ailment | Symptoms | Remedy |
|---|---|---|
| Anxiety with a lack of confidence | Apprehension about public performance; inability to sleep for reviewing day's events. | *Lycopodium* see p.31 |
| Anxiety with restlessness | Chilliness; tiredness; appetite disturbance; clammy skin, fast pulse; tidy and fastidious. | *Arsen. alb.* see p.37 |
| Anxiety relieved by reassurance | Nervousness; sensitivity to others, but wanting limelight; fear of many things like dark. | *Phos.* see p.44 |

## 83 ANGER

Along with irritability, this is a natural response to events that seem threatening or frightening. There may be physical symptoms *(see right)*, and it can be caused by overwork, too much food and alcohol, tiredness, or fear of coming events. Exercise helps with anger and irritability.

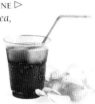

EXTREME ANGER ▷
*Anger may be accompanied by a fast pulse, stomach flutters, and muscle tension.*

# 84 TIREDNESS & INSOMNIA

Tiredness is usually due to lack of sleep, physical or emotional stress, or overwork, although it can be related to anaemia or other vitamin or mineral deficiencies. Common tiredness responds to rest and extra sleep; vitamin and mineral supplements may also help. Insomnia can be due to too many late nights, stress, food allergy, or depression, and results in severe exhaustion and disturbed sleep patterns: difficulty getting to sleep and frequent waking. If it does not improve in three weeks, see a doctor.

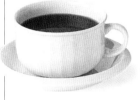

◁ STIMULANTS
*Excess caffeine can cause insomnia, as can alcohol, food allergy, stress, anxiety, or depression. Avoid eating late at night.*

△ RELAXING ROUTINE
*An hour before bedtime, drink a herbal tea, have a warm bath, and read something light to wind down before trying to sleep.*

# 85 SHOCK & BEREAVEMENT

Shock is a reaction to a frightening or upsetting event, or can follow an injury. If it is accompanied by nausea and vomiting, fainting or clouding of consciousness, call an ambulance. *Gelsemium (see p.28)* and *Aconite (see p.22)* benefit people in shock.

Bereavement has four stages lasting over a few years: numb disbelief; denial; anger or guilt that not enough was done; and fading depression. It is helped in the early stages by *Arnica (see p.24)*, *Aconite (see p.22)*, and *Ignatia (see p.30)*.

# 86 DEPRESSION

This includes a wide range of feelings from sadness to total despair. Where there is a specific cause such as hormonal problem (like postnatal depression) or after a viral infection, it tends to disappear in time. Sometimes there is no specific cause, and it lingers. If this is the case, see a doctor.

PASQUE FLOWER ▷
*The homeopathic remedy made from this plant is* Pulsatilla. *It is used in the treatment of very tearful depression.*

# DIGESTIVE DISORDERS

## 87 INDIGESTION

This term describes various symptoms brought on by eating: stomach-ache, heartburn, nausea, and excessive flatulence and burping. Relax before eating, eat slowly, and avoid eating late.

△ SPICY FOOD
*Fatty, spicy, rich foods can cause indigestion.*

| AILMENT | SYMPTOMS | REMEDY |
| --- | --- | --- |
| Indigestion with excessive flatulence | Digestion seems slower; even plain foods cause pain; headache; burning in stomach. | *Carbo veg.* *see p.39* |
| Indigestion with painful retching | Overwrought from stress; irritability; heartburn; craving for fatty, sour, or spicy foods. | *Nux vomica* *see p.32* |
| Indigestion with nausea and vomiting | Begins two hours after eating; pressure under breastbone; pounding heart; headache. | *Pulsatilla* *see p.33* |

## 88 BLOATING & FLATULENCE

These can be caused by constipation, premenstrual tension, swallowing air when you eat, food intolerance, or nervous apprehension. Certain foods exacerbate flatulence and bloating; where possible avoid eating pulses, onions, cabbage, and nuts.

| AILMENT | SYMPTOMS | REMEDY |
| --- | --- | --- |
| Bloating after eating only small amounts of food | Impossible to pass stools without straining; release of flatulence provides no relief. | *Lycopodium* *see p.31* |
| Bloating and flatulence relieved by burping | Burning in stomach and much flatulence; aversion to meat and milk; crave salt. | *Carbo veg.* *see p.39* |

# 89 VOMITING & NAUSEA

Nausea and vomiting may be due to an infection; migraine; stress; too much food or alcohol; contaminated food or water; gall-bladder or liver disorders; hormone changes; or inner ear problems. For severe abdominal pain or vomited blood, call an ambulance.

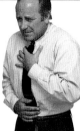

◁ VOMITING
*If vomiting persists for more than 48 hours, and/or there is blood in the stools, see a doctor, within two hours, if possible.*

| AILMENT | SYMPTOMS | REMEDY |
|---|---|---|
| Constant nausea | Nausea not relieved by vomiting; may have diarrhoea and headache; much saliva. | *Ipecac.* *see p.30* |
| Vomiting with great thirst | Great thirst, but drinks are vomited; burning pain with retching and vomiting. | *Phos.* *see p.44* |
| Nausea and vomiting with weepiness | Weepiness, depression, desire for sympathy; may be mucus dripping down throat. | *Pulsatilla* *see p.33* |

# 90 DIARRHOEA & CONSTIPATION

Constipation is usually caused by a diet too low in fibre, although tension and a sedentary lifestyle may contribute. Diarrhoea is a symptom of gastroenteritis, but is also associated with food allergy or intolerance, and stress, and can be a side effect of certain drugs. If there is bleeding from the anus, see a doctor within 12 hours.

◁ ALOE VERA
Aloe, *made from aloe vera leaves, is used to treat diarrhoea that results from food intolerance.*

| AILMENT | SYMPTOMS | REMEDY |
|---|---|---|
| Diarrhoea from nervous excitement | Accompanied by flatulence; greenish stools; craving for sweet, salty, and cold foods. | *Argentum nit.* *see p.36* |
| Diarrhoea with irritation of skin round anus | Urgent need to pass stools early in the morning; possible piles. | *Sulphur* *see p.45* |
| Constipation caused by sluggish bowels | No desire to open bowels until rectum is full; stools soft or covered in mucus. | *Alumina* Ask your homeopath for details of this remedy. |

# 91 URINARY DISORDERS

In homeopathy, urinary disorders are viewed not just as problems in the kidneys and urinary system, but as a mirror of the body's functioning and diet. Stress increases chemicals in the body, which must be excreted, while a poor diet strains the whole metabolism and the kidneys in particular. To prevent urinary disorders, avoid too much stress, eat sensibly, exercise, and drink plenty of fluids to cleanse the kidneys.

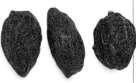

△ SAW PALMETTO
*The Sabal remedy is made from the berries and seeds of the saw palmetto, and is given for an enlarged prostate gland, and testicular inflammation.*

Cystitis is caused by infection or by an irritiation of the bladder. It results in painful urination, with increased frequency. Without treatment it can develop into a serious kidney infection.

In stress incontinence, trickles of urine are passed involuntarily as a result of coughing, sneezing, laughing, or lifting. It is caused by weakened pelvic floor muscles.

PRECAUTIONS
• *Cystitis: if there is pain in the kidneys or blood in the urine, see a doctor. Never supress the urge to urinate.*
• *Prostate enlargement: prostate problems should always be referred to a doctor. The cause is unknown, although they are common in men over 45.*
• *Stress incontinence: to strengthen pelvic floor muscles, tighten then relax them.*

| AILMENT | SYMPTOMS | REMEDY |
|---|---|---|
| Cystitis with a non-stop desire to urinate | Burning, cutting pain in lower abdomen; little urine, with some blood in it. | *Cantharis* *see p.19* |
| Cystitis with painful urging | Despite frequent need to urinate, very little is passed; chilliness; irritability. | *Nux vomica* *see p.32* |
| Cystitis with a continuous burning sensation | Sensation that a drop of urine is constantly trickling through; resentfulness. | *Staphysagria* Ask your homeopath for details of this remedy. |
| Enlarged prostate with a constant desire to urinate | Urination difficult; possible penile discharge; spasms in bladder or urethra. | *Sabal* *see above* |
| Involuntary leakage of urine | Urine leaks unnoticed when pressure in the abdomen rises, e.g. when coughing. | *Causticum* Ask your homeopath for details of this remedy. |

# FIRST AID

## 92 FIRST AID KIT

Homeopathic remedies can play an important part in accidents and emergencies, especially the treatment of minor flesh wounds. Their purpose is to ease pain, calm the mind, and help the body to heal itself. Keep a homeopathic first aid kit, such as the one below for minor injuries, but in serious accidents, get expert help as soon as possible. Store the kit in a dark, cool place away from children.

FIRST AID REMEDIES ▽
*For acute first aid complaints, use a dosage of 30c potency, for less acute use 6c. These are safe for babies, children, and adults.*

*Tablets to have a supply of include Apis 30c; Bryonia 30c; Cantharis 6c, 30c; Euphrasia 6c; Glonoin. 30c; Hypericum 30c; Ledum 6c; Nux vomica 6c; Phos. 6c; Rhus tox. 6c; Ruta grav. 6c; Silicea 6c; Tabacum 6c; and Urtica 6c.*

*Bandages and sterile dressings should be included in the kit as well.*

*Homeopathic tinctures are the same as herbal tinctures, and can be bought ready-made. Keep tinctures of Arnica, Calendula, Hypericum, Euphrasia, and Pyrethrum.*

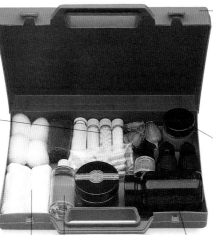

*A sturdy case or box for storage is essential. If kept in a cool, dark, dry place remedies will last for years.*

*Creams and ointments can be bought ready made. Keep Arnica cream and Calendula cream, and Urtica ointment.*

*Arnica is the most valuable remedy in the first aid kit. Available in tablet, cream, or tincture form, it steadies the nerves, and reduces swelling and bruises.*

# 93 CUTS & GRAZES

If a cut or graze bleeds, infection may occur, and there may be bruising. Clean the wound with a calendula and hypericum solution. Cover with a sterile dressing to prevent infection.

◁ ARNICA CREAM
*The cream form of this excellent first aid remedy should never be applied to skin that is broken.*

| CUTS & GRAZES | REMEDY | | DOSAGE |
|---|---|---|---|
| Wound has moderate to severe bruising | *Arnica see p.24* | | 30c every 2 hours for 6 doses, then 3 times a day for 6 days. |
| Wound feels numb and cold | *Ledum see p.31* Apply cold compress to soothe. | | 30c every 2 hours for 6 doses, then 3 times a day for 6 days. |
| Wound with shooting nerve pain | *Hypericum see p.29* Leave dressing in place for 2–3 days. | | 30c every 2 hours for up to 3 days. |

# 94 BURNS & SCALDS

Burns are most common in children and older people; many are due to accidents in the home, which are usually preventable. Minor burns and scalds are painful: avoid touching them more than necessary. Immerse the wound in cold running water to cool the skin and reduce pain. Apply urtica ointment to soothe superficial burns. If a burn is bigger than the palm of your hand, you should see a doctor.

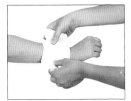

APPLYING URTICA
*Once you have applied the ointment, cover the burn with a sterile dressing.*

| BURNS AND SCALDS | REMEDY | | DOSAGE |
|---|---|---|---|
| Burn may form a blister; searing smarting pain | *Arnica see p.24* Followed by: *Cantharis see p.19* ▷  Soothe burns and scalds with a cold compress. | | 30c every 15 minutes for up to 3 doses. then 30c every 15 minutes for up to 6 doses. |
| Continuous stinging pain | *Urtica see p.35* | | 6c every 15 minutes for up to 10 doses. |

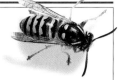

# 95 INSECT STINGS

Insect stings cause pain, swelling, and sometimes, infection. If a sting is inside the mouth, rinse out the mouth with iced water to prevent any swelling, and see a doctor. If there is any sign of an allergic reation, seek medical attention.

Remove bee and wasp stings with sterilized tweezers. Apply pyrethrum tincture to the sting.

**TREATING STINGS △**
*Soothe stings in the first instance by applying pyrethrum tincture.*

| INSECT STINGS | REMEDY | DOSAGE |
|---|---|---|
| Sting is swollen, bruised, and painful | Arnica see p.24 Followed by: Ledum see p.31 If a sting is inside the mouth, rinse with iced water to stop swelling, and see a doctor. | 30c every 5 minutes for up to 10 doses then 6c every 8 hours for up to 3 days. |
| Sting is hot, red, and painful | Apis see p.18 | 30c every 15 minutes for up to 6 doses. |

# 96 NOSE BLEEDS

These can occur after an injury to the nose or can be brought on by blowing the nose violently. To stop bleeding, sit down with the head well forward, with the mouth held open, and pinch the lower part of the nostrils firmly for ten minutes. The sufferer should breathe through the mouth. The nostrils should then be released slowly, and the sufferer should avoid touching or blowing the nose. If bleeding persists, you should seek medical attention.

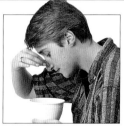

**STOPPING THE BLEEDING**
*Place a bowl on the table in front of you to catch any stray drips that may fall.*

| NOSEBLEEDS | REMEDY | DOSAGE |
|---|---|---|
| Nosebleed that occurs after an injury | Arnica see p.24 | 6c every 2 minutes for up to 10 doses. |
| Nosebleed from blowing nose violently | Phos. see p.44 | 6c every 2 minutes for up to 10 doses. |

# 97 HEAT EXHAUSTION

This is caused by excessive fluid loss in hot, humid weather, and interferes with the control of blood circulation to the head and heart. Symptoms include sudden flushes of heat due to increased blood flow up to the head.

Lay the person who is suffering in a cool place. Give frequent sips of salty water. To make the salt solution, add 5ml (1 teaspoon) of salt per 1 litre (1¼ pints) of water.

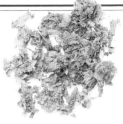

△ BRYONY PULPED ROOT
*Fresh bryony root is pulped to make the homeopathic remedy.*

| HEAT EXHAUSTION | REMEDY | DOSAGE |
|---|---|---|
| Severe headache worse for moving; nausea | *Bryonia see p.25* Symptoms are better for plenty of rest. | 30c every 5 minutes for up to 10 doses. |
| Throbbing headache; hot face; sweaty | *Glonoin.* Ask a homeopath for more details. | 30c every 5 minutes for up to 10 doses. |

# 98 TRAVEL SICKNESS

Motion sickness, or travel sickness, occurs when the balance mechanism of the inner ear is upset by the movement of a car, boat, train, or aeroplane. Children are particularly vulnerable.

Symptoms come on suddenly and can include excessive saliva, pain, chilliness with perspiration, anxiety and vertigo. They are aggravated by the slightest motion, and improve when motion ceases.

Homeopathic remedies can be taken one hour before starting a journey to prevent the onset of travel sickness.

TOBACCO △
Tabacum *remedy is made from tobacco leaves.*

| TRAVEL SICKNESS | REMEDY | DOSAGE |
|---|---|---|
| Nausea; giddiness and faintness; sweating | *Tabacum see above* | 6c every 15 minutes for up to 10 doses. |
| Queasiness; chilliness; headache | *Nux vomica see p.32* | 6c every 15 minutes for up to 10 doses. |

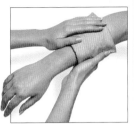

# 99 SPRAINS & STRAINS

Over-stretching the ligaments (the fibres that bind the joints together) causes sprains. Strains, also caused by over-stretching, affect the muscles. Treat both with ten doses of *Arnica* followed by *Ruta grav.* for sprains, and *Rhus tox.* for strains. Symptoms of both include swelling and pain whenever the joint or muscle is used.

1 ▷ Add 10 drops of arnica tincture to a bowl of cold water and soak a cold compress in it. Wring the compress out, ready for use. In the meantime, support the injured joint or muscle as comfortably as possible.

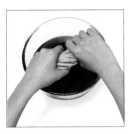

2 △ Apply the cold arnica compress to the affected area to reduce swelling. If the ankle is sprained, apply arnica cream and bandage firmly. If pain and swelling are not relieved by this homeopathic treatment see a doctor.

# 100 BLISTERS

Blisters are bubbles of fluid that form under the skin. They can be caused as a result of either friction or burns. If a blister bursts, bathe it with a solution of calendula and hypericum, made by adding 10 drops each of *Calendula* tincture and *Hypericum* tincture to 1.25 litres (2 pints) of cooled boiled water.
• For burning, itchy blisters, apply a cold compress to the affected part and take 6c *Cantharis* four times a day until the pain wears off.
• If the blister is extremely itchy, red, and swollen, then take a 6c dose of *Rhus tox.* four times a day until the pain subsides.

# 101 SPLINTERS

A sharp-edged piece of wood, stone, or metal that breaks off under the skin can cause an infection. In the first instance, remove the splinter with tweezers that you have sterilized. The stinging, burning pain will be relieved by a warm compress, which may also help to draw deeply embedded splinters to the surface. Take a 6c dose of *Silicea* four times a day for up to 14 days.

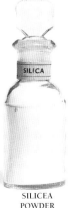

SILICEA
POWDER

# INDEX

# ACKNOWLEDGMENTS

**Dorling Kindersley** would like to thank:
Hilary Bird for compiling the index;
Marshall Baron for proof reading;
Susie Behar for editorial assistance;
and Robert Campbell for DTP assistance.

**Photography**
KEY: t *top*; b *bottom*; c *centre*; l *left*; r *right*
All photography by Andy Crawford and Steve Gorton except for:
Brian Cosgrove: 8 cr; GeoScience Features Picture Library:
Dr B. Booth 44 tc; NHPA: Jany Sauvanet 20 c;
Science Photo Library: Vaughan Fleming 42 cl.

Text from this book originally appeared in
*The Complete Guide to Homeopathy*,
published by Dorling Kindersley Ltd. 1995.